Trauma, Repair and Recovery

Edited by James Phillips

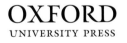

The Open University

OXFORD
UNIVERSITY PRESS

Published by Oxford University Press, Great Clarendon Street, Oxford OX2 6DP
in association with The Open University, Walton Hall, Milton Keynes MK7 6AA.

Oxford University Press is a department of the University of Oxford. It furthers the University's
objective of excellence in research, scholarship, and education by publishing worldwide in

Oxford New York
Auckland Cape Town Dar es Salaam Hong Kong Karachi Kuala Lumpur Madrid Melbourne
Mexico City Nairobi New Delhi Shanghai Taipei Toronto

with offices in
Argentina Austria Brazil Chile Czech Republic France Greece Guatemala Hungary
Italy Japan Poland Portugal Singapore South Korea Switzerland
Thailand Turkey Ukraine Vietnam

Oxford is a registered trade mark of Oxford University Press in the UK and in certain
other countries.

Published in the United States by Oxford University Press Inc., New York

First published 2008

Edited and designed by The Open University.

Typeset by SR Nova Pvt. Ltd, Bangalore, India.

Printed and bound in the United Kingdom at the University Press, Cambridge.

This book forms part of the Open University course SDK125 *Introducing Health Sciences: A Case
Study Approach*. Details of this and other Open University courses can be obtained from the Student
Registration and Enquiry Service, The Open University, PO Box 197, Milton Keynes MK7 6BJ,
United Kingdom:
tel. +44 (0)870 333 4340, email general-enquiries@open.ac.uk.

http://www.open.ac.uk

British Library Cataloguing in Publication Data available on request

Library of Congress Cataloging in Publication Data available on request

ISBN 9780 1992 3734 0

10 9 8 7 6 5 4 3 2 1

ABOUT THIS BOOK

This book and the accompanying material on DVD present the sixth case study in a series of seven, under the collective title *Introducing Health Sciences: A Case Study Approach*. Together they form an Open University (OU) course for students beginning the first year of an undergraduate programme in Health Sciences. Each case study has also been designed to 'stand alone' for readers studying it in isolation from the rest of the course, either as part of an educational programme at another institution, or for general interest and self-directed study.

Trauma, Repair and Recovery is a multidisciplinary introduction to the important health topic of how the human body responds to trauma. Traumatic injury is a leading cause of death and disability throughout the world and is likely to remain so in future years, particularly as road traffic increases. The incidence of traumatic injury at a global level is considered, and case descriptions illustrate the nature of damage and repair and its impact on the people affected. In particular, this book focuses on the tissue-level biology of the human body, comparing and contrasting how different tissues are structured, how they interact with each other during normal physiology and how they repair following damage. The initial life-threatening issues that can follow trauma are reviewed, and the assessment of damage, treatment and long-term recovery are described. Trauma can be mental as well as physical; occasionally the psychological harm is long-lasting and for some people may be more disabling than the physical injury. The mechanisms that give rise to these distressing symptoms will be discussed, together with the sorts of treatment available.

No previous experience of studying science has been assumed and new concepts and specialist terminology are explained with examples and illustrations. There is some straightforward mathematical content, including some interpretation of data in tables and graphs, and a small section on calculating forces.

To help you plan your study of this material, we have included a number of 'icons' in the margin to indicate different types of activity which have been included to help you develop and practise particular skills. This icon indicates when to undertake an activity on the accompanying DVD. You will need to 'run' the DVD programs on your computer because they are *interactive,* and this function doesn't operate on a domestic DVD-player. The DVD has six sequences: a short film made by the World Health Organization entitled 'Road safety is no accident'; a video of UK paramedics dealing with a simulated road traffic collision, which concludes with an interactive exercise demonstrating the effects of shock on heart rate and blood pressure; two videos in which people describe how their lives have been affected by traumatic injuries, and two interactive 3D animations showing how the tissues in a 'virtual' leg are arranged and summarising the repair sequences of each tissue.

Activities involving pencil-and-paper exercises are indicated by this icon, and if you need a calculator you will see . Some additional activities for Open University students only are described in a *Companion* text, which is not available outside the OU course. These are indicated by this icon in the margin. Some activities involve using the internet and are marked by this icon . References to activities for OU students are given in the margins of the

v

book and should not interrupt your concentration if you are not studying it as part of an OU course.

At various points in the book, you will find 'boxed' material of two types: Explanation Boxes and Enrichment Boxes. The Explanation Boxes contain basic concepts explained in the kind of detail that someone who is completely new to the health sciences is likely to want. The Enrichment Boxes contain extension material, included for added interest, particularly if you already have some knowledge of basic science. If you are studying this book as part of an OU course, you should note that the Explanation Boxes contain material that is *essential* to your learning and which therefore may be *assessed*. However, the content of the Enrichment Boxes will *not* be tested in the course assessments.

The authors' intention is to bring you into the subject, develop confidence through activities and guidance, and provide a stepping stone into further study. The most important terms appear in **bold** font in the text at the point where they are first defined, and these terms are also in bold in the index at the end of the book. Understanding of the meaning and uses of the bold terms is essential (i.e. assessable) if you are an OU student.

Active engagement with the material throughout this book is encouraged by numerous 'in text' questions, indicated by a diamond symbol (◆), followed immediately by our suggested answers. It is good practice always to cover the answer and attempt your own response to the question before reading ours. At the end of each chapter, there is a summary of the key points and a list of the main learning outcomes, followed by self-assessment questions to enable you to test your own learning. The answers to these questions are at the back of the book. The great majority of the learning outcomes should be achievable by anyone who has studied this book and its DVD material; one or two learning outcomes for some chapters are only achievable by OU students who have completed the *Companion* activities, and these are clearly identified.

Internet database (ROUTES)

A large amount of valuable information is available via the internet. To help OU students and other readers of books in this series to access good quality sites without having to search for hours, the OU has developed a collection of internet resources on a searchable database called ROUTES. All websites included in the database are selected by academic staff or subject-specialist librarians. The content of each website is evaluated to ensure that it is accurate, well presented and regularly updated. A description is included for each of the resources.

The website address for ROUTES is: http://routes.open.ac.uk/

Entering the Open University course code 'SDK125' in the search box will retrieve all the resources that have been recommended for this book. Alternatively, if you want to search for any resources on a particular subject, type in the words that best describe the subject you are interested in (for example, 'trauma'), or browse the alphabetical list of subjects.

Authors' acknowledgements

As ever in The Open University, this book and DVD combine the efforts of many people with specialist skills and knowledge in different disciplines. The principal authors were James Phillips (biology), Jeanne Katz and Tom Heller (health and social care), Jamie Harle (physics), Peter Naish (psychology) and Basiro Davey (public health). Our contributions have been shaped and immeasurably enriched by the OU course team who helped us to plan the content and made numerous comments and suggestions for improvements as the material progressed through several drafts. It would be impossible to thank everyone personally, but we would like to acknowledge the help and support of academic colleagues who have contributed to this book (in alphabetical order of discipline): Nicolette Habgood, Heather McLannahan, Carol Midgley, Hilary MacQueen (biology), Lesley Smart (chemistry), Elizabeth Parvin (physics) and Frederick Toates (psychology).

The multimedia animations on the DVD were produced by Autonomy Multimedia Ltd, and in the OU by Steve Best and Greg Black (LTS) and Brian Richardson (SWIM team). The audiovisual material was developed by Owen Horn and Jo Mack (Sound and Vision), with James Phillips, Hilary MacQueen, Jeanne Katz, Peter Naish and Basiro Davey.

We are very grateful to our External Assessor, Professor Susan Standring, Head of the Department of Anatomy and Human Sciences, Kings College London, whose detailed comments have contributed to the structure and content of the book and the anatomical material on the DVD, and kept the needs of our intended readership to the fore. We also acknowledge the valuable contribution made by our external critical reader, Dr Rosalind Phillips (GP Registrar).

Special thanks are due to all those involved in the OU production process, chief among them Joy Wilson and Dawn Partner, our wonderful Course Manager and Course Team Assistant, whose commitment, efficiency and unflagging good humour were at the heart of the endeavour. We also warmly acknowledge the contributions of our editor, Bina Sharma, whose skill has improved every aspect of this book; Steve Best, our graphic artist, who developed and drew all the diagrams; Sarah Hofton and Chris Hough, our graphic designers, who devised the page designs and layouts; and Martin Keeling, who carried out picture research and rights clearance. The activity to support Open University students in developing their information literacy was devised by Clari Hunt (OU Library). The media project managers were Judith Pickering and James Davies.

For the copublication process, we would especially like to thank Jonathan Crowe of Oxford University Press and, from within The Open University, Christianne Bailey (Media Developer, Copublishing). As is the custom, any small errors or shortcomings that have slipped in (despite our collective best efforts) remain the responsibility of the authors. We would be pleased to receive feedback on the book (favourable or otherwise). Please write to the address below.

Dr Basiro Davey, SDK125 Course Team Chair

Department of Biological Sciences
The Open University
Walton Hall
Milton Keynes
MK7 6AA
United Kingdom

Environmental statement

Paper and board used in this publication is FSC certified.

Forestry Stewardship Council (FSC) is an independent certification, which certifies that the virgin pulp used to make the paper/board comes from traceable and sustainable sources from well-managed forests.

CONTENTS

The DVD activities associated with this book were written, designed and developed by Autonomy Multimedia Ltd, Steve Best, Greg Black, Basiro Davey, Owen Horn, Jo Mack, Hilary MacQueen and James Phillips.

CHAPTER 1

TRAUMATIC INJURY IN THE 'HUMAN ZOO'

1.1 Introduction

This book takes a health sciences approach to the subject of **trauma** – a term that encompasses any physical injury or a severe psychological shock. Where it is important to distinguish these two meanings, we will refer to **traumatic injury** to the body and **psychological trauma**. Trauma is a neglected public-health problem of immense global importance, rising year by year as urbanisation crowds over half the world's population into the equivalent of 'human zoos'. Over 5 million people die every year as a result of accidental or intentional traumatic injuries (that's almost 16 000 a day) and around half a billion survivors suffer a physical or psychological trauma as a result.

Road crashes are one cause of trauma where the rate of fatalities is falling in many of the world's richest countries, but is increasing rapidly in most developing countries (Figure 1.1) where more than 80% of the world's population live. Following present trends, traffic-related injuries are predicted to rise from almost 1.2 million in 2002 to 2.1 million by 2030 – a prediction that led the World Health Organization (WHO) to devote its 2004 World Health Day to road safety (Figure 1.2). But traffic accidents are

The health effects of living in the 'human zoo' are reviewed in another book in this series, *Water and Health in an Overcrowded World* (Halliday and Davey, 2007).

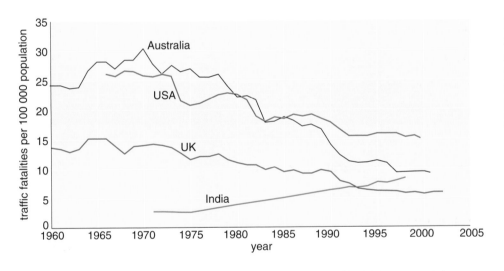

Figure 1.1 Trends in traffic-related mortality in India, Australia, the USA and the UK per 100 000 population, from the 1960s to the late 1990s. (Source: data from Peden et al., 2004, Figures 2.4 and 2.5, p. 38)

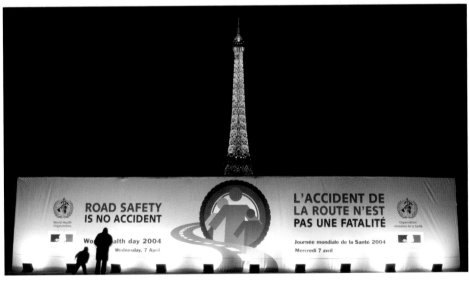

Figure 1.2 A giant banner before the Eiffel Tower in Paris advertises the World Health Organization's 'World Health Day', 7 April 2004, highlighting the global challenge of traffic-related injuries. (Source: WHO)

far from being the only increasing cause of trauma: interpersonal violence and self-inflicted harm are increasing almost everywhere, prompting the WHO to establish its Department of Injuries and Violence Prevention in 2000.

Most people will know of someone who has had a serious accident or other trauma. However, most people are unaware of what a large and increasing contribution trauma makes to deaths and disabilities worldwide. This chapter describes the global **epidemiology** of trauma – the occurrence, distribution and control of disability and death from traumatic injuries in different populations. We focus most attention on traffic crashes because they are the single largest cause of injuries worldwide, and the nature of the injuries arising from road accidents and their immediate and longer-term consequences are discussed in detail later in the book.

Chapter 2 looks at some of the immediate medical responses to life-threatening traumatic injury; then Chapter 3 explores the structure of the body tissues most frequently damaged during trauma. Fractures are discussed in Chapter 4, with a focus on falls in older people, before Chapter 5 explains the science of tissue repair and how the nature of the tissue that is damaged influences the extent of recovery. Finally, Chapter 6 looks at the long-term consequences of trauma, including a discussion of post-traumatic stress disorder (PTSD) and the global costs of traffic accidents. Throughout, we emphasise that a multidisciplinary approach is required to understand how traumatic injury affects individuals physically and psychologically.

As this book progresses, we will illustrate the effect of trauma on human lives through a series of case descriptions or 'vignettes'. Each vignette is set within a specific culture and geographical region but you should recognise that there will be similarities and differences between the chosen examples and people with other characteristics, or from other parts of the world.

1.2   Variations in the risk of death from injury

The types of events that cause traumatic injuries are distributed unevenly between different parts of the world, between males and females and in different age-groups. This section briefly reviews variations in the risks of dying from accidental or intentional injuries.

The actual number of road traffic deaths given in WHO statistics is 1 191 796 (see Table 1.1); this is often 'rounded up' and expressed as the decimal number '1.2 million' (one million, two-hundred thousand).

Worldwide, road-traffic injuries account for the largest share of trauma-related deaths – almost 23% of the total in 2002 (Figure 1.3). In that year, road crashes killed almost 1.2 million people. The next largest category, 'other unintentional injuries', includes deaths due to natural disasters and accidents other than falls, fires, drowning and poisoning (the categories routinely reported in WHO statistics).

◆ According to Figure 1.3, which category of *intentional* injuries contributed the highest proportion to trauma-related deaths in 2002?

◆ The fact that almost 17% of all trauma-related deaths were due to self-inflicted injuries may have surprised you. Suicides exceed the combined total of deaths due to interpersonal violence, warfare and other intentional injuries.

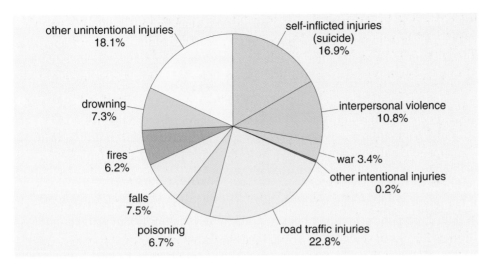

Figure 1.3 A 'pie chart' showing the percentage of global deaths from trauma due to major causes of injury in 2002. (Source: data from Peden et al., 2004, Figure 2.1, p. 34)

1.2.1 Variations by region

The map in Figure 1.4 illustrates regional variations in **mortality rates** due to traumatic injury in the year 2000, i.e. the number of injury-related deaths that year, expressed as a *rate* per 100 000 population in each region.

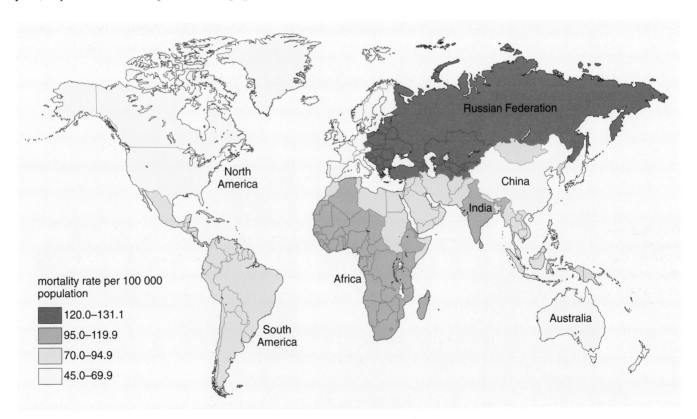

Figure 1.4 Trauma-related mortality rates (per 100 000 population) in different regions of the world in 2000. (Source: WHO, 2002, un-numbered diagram, p. 11)

◆ Why would comparing the total *number* of injury-related deaths in different countries or regions give a misleading impression of their relative importance and how does expressing the data as a *rate* overcome this problem?

◆ A larger number of injury-related deaths will inevitably occur in larger populations than in smaller ones, so just comparing the *number* of deaths may create a false impression that injury is a bigger health problem in large populations. Expressing deaths as a *rate* per 100 000 people in each population allows direct comparisons of the rates of injury in countries or regions with different population sizes.

It is a neglected truth that less than 20% of the 5 million deaths from all types of injury that occur each year happen in the high-income 'developed' countries (principally Western Europe, North America, Japan, Australia and New Zealand). As Figure 1.4 shows, the relatively less affluent countries of Eastern Europe and the former Union of Soviet Socialist Republics have the highest trauma-related mortality rates of anywhere in the world, with the rates in most of Africa and South-East Asia not far behind. The reasons for higher death rates from injury in low- and middle-income countries are complex and we do not have space to discuss them in detail here, but they include:

- More hazardous conditions in the workplace, in homes and in public places (e.g. unsafe equipment and working practices, faulty electrical wiring, crumbling infrastructure, unguarded stairways, etc.).

- Rapidly increasing traffic congestion.

- Larger numbers of pedestrians and higher proportions of two-wheeled vehicles, whose passengers are particularly vulnerable (Figure 1.5).

- Overcrowding in public transport, so larger numbers of people are killed or injured in any crash.

- Relatively low safety standards in the maintenance of vehicles and roads, poor enforcement of traffic-safety regulations, inadequate traffic control and few measures to protect pedestrians (Figure 1.6).

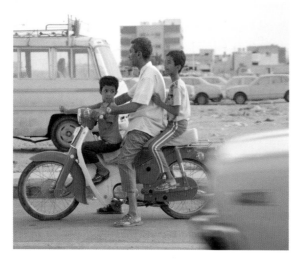

Figure 1.5 Overloaded two-wheeled motorcycles and bikes are frequently involved in traffic accidents in developing countries. (Source: Ralph Henning/Alamy)

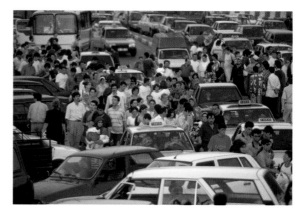

Figure 1.6 Rush-hour traffic and pedestrians mingle in Istanbul, Turkey. (Source: Mark Henley/Panos Pictures)

- Higher rates of interpersonal violence and warfare.

- Higher rates of poverty, unemployment and discrimination leading to higher rates of suicide and self-harm.

- Patterns of alcohol consumption that typically involve 'binge' drinking of vodka and illegally distilled spirits, which greatly increases the risk of accidental or self-inflicted injury and violence.

- Limited health services to treat injuries, compounded by lack of ambulances and paramedics to transport seriously injured people to hospital.

Alcohol and Human Health is the subject of another book in this series (Smart, 2007).

1.2.2 Variations by age-group

The total number of deaths worldwide in each of the trauma categories is given in Table 1.1 for different age groups in 2002. The rank position of each cause relative to all causes of death in that year is shown in brackets. For example, if you look along the row labelled 'road traffic accidents (RTAs)', you can see from the first column that they caused the deaths of 50 139 children aged 0–4 years worldwide in 2002, and that RTAs ranked 13th among all causes of death in this age-group in that year.

Table 1.1 Leading causes of death due to injuries in 2002 by age-group, both sexes combined, and (in brackets) the worldwide ranking as a cause of all deaths in that age-group. (Source: data derived from Global Burden of Disease Project, 2002, revised Statistical Annex)

Cause of injury	0–4 years	5–14 years	15–29 years	30–44 years	45–59 years	60+ years	All ages
Unintentional injuries	288 526	371 175	766 223	707 566	618 379	798 704	3 550 573
road traffic accidents (RTAs)	50 139 (13)	132 695 (2)	304 994 (2)	287 730 (3)	222 249 (8)	193 990 (22)	1 191 796 (11)
poisoning	15 647 (26)	19 982 (13)	51 494 (12)	81 678 (10)	99 803 (19)	81 760 (36)	350 365 (29)
falls	16 438 (23)	20 580 (12)	37 874 (15)	45 068 (19)	60 920 (26)	210 883 (19)	391 764 (27)
fires	39 669 (16)	34 180 (7)	89 130 (8)	64 494 (12)	37 103 (34)	46 960 (42)	311 534 (33)
drowning	57 973 (12)	86 953 (4)	89 196 (7)	58 725 (14)	44 074 (31)	45 391 (43)	382 312 (28)
other unintentional	108 661	76 785	193 535	169 872	154 230	219 719	922 802
Intentional injuries	13 820	36 007	541 783	460 400	304 891	260 842	1 617 742
self-inflicted	120 (66)	14 762 (16)	251 446 (3)	230 997 (5)	187 696 (9)	188 340 (23)	873 361 (15)
interpersonal violence	12 618 (31)	18 340 (14)	216 648 (5)	166 661 (6)	91 145 (20)	53 958 (39)	559 370 (22)
war injuries	364 (62)	2244 (38)	69 707 (9)	59 359 (13)	24 142 (42)	16 363 (57)	172 180 (46)
other intentional	718	661	3982	3383	1908	2180	12 831
ALL injuries	302 345	407 183	1 308 005	1 167 966	923 270	1 059 546	5 168 315

If you look along the bottom row of Table 1.1 and do some addition, you will find that almost half of all injury-related deaths occur between the ages of 15 and 44 years (2 475 971 deaths, compared with 2 692 344 in all other age groups combined). This statistic has profound consequences for the families of those who die, over and above the emotional loss.

◆ Can you suggest why?

◆ This age-group includes the main wage-earning years in many populations, particularly in developing countries: the death of a wage-earner has long-term financial implications for families and can tip those on low incomes into poverty. (We return to this subject at the end of the book.)

There are two reasons for caution before considering the data in Table 1.1 in more detail. The first is that there are bound to be inaccuracies in the numbers of deaths reported to the WHO in each trauma category, depending on the quality of the death registration system and other sources of injury-related data in each country (e.g. police records of accidents, hospital statistics, research surveys and reports from 'victim-support' and other voluntary organisations).

◆ The level of inaccuracy is bound to be greatest in countries with the least resources for data collection. Do you think that the reported trauma statistics for these countries are likely to be under- or over-estimates, and why?

◆ Countries that cannot afford to collect systematic data on deaths and assign them to a particular cause are likely to *under*-estimate the total because a substantial number of cases will be missed from the records. Accidents in remote or rural areas and among the poorest sections of any society are less likely to be reported to the authorities.

The second reason for caution relates to the meaning attached to the *ranking* of trauma-related deaths in each age-group. Table 1.1 shows that in 2002, deaths from road traffic accidents were the second highest cause of death globally in the age-groups 5–14 and 15–29 years and the third highest cause among 30–44 year-olds. Deaths due to traffic would rank *even higher* in these age groups if it wasn't for the huge increase in deaths from HIV/AIDS since the 1980s. Traffic-related deaths have been pushed *lower* in the ranking even though the total number of deaths from this cause is *rising*. Categories can change ranking (up or down) from year to year, depending on fluctuations in *other* causes of death. Notice too that the absolute *number* of deaths from a particular cause doesn't enable you to predict its ranking.

◆ Look at the *number* of deaths from drowning in the age-groups 5–14 and 15–29 years and compare this with the *ranking* of drowning as a cause of death in each age-group. What do you notice?

◆ Around 87 000 people drowned in the 5–14 age-group in 2002, and drowning was ranked the 4th highest cause of all deaths among 5–14 year-olds that year; there were 2000 *more* drownings among 15–29 year-olds, but this ranked 7th among their causes of death.

◆ Can you see from Table 1.1 why drowning is ranked lower as a cause of death among 15–29 year-olds, even though 2000 more people died than in the 5–14 year-olds?

◆ The drop in ranking is at least partly because this age group suffers many more self-inflicted deaths and deaths from interpersonal violence and fires than among 5–14 year-olds, which 'pushes' drownings down the rank order.

Among the youngest age-group (0–4 years), drowning is ranked the 12th highest cause of *all* deaths and the commonest cause of *injury-related* deaths worldwide. Among older people, deaths from injuries are a neglected topic, submerged in the rank order by cardiovascular disease, cancers and respiratory conditions such as chronic obstructive pulmonary disease (COPD). In 2002, there were 1 059 546 injury-related deaths in people aged 60 years and over. As Table 1.1 shows, a somewhat larger number of older people died as a result of a fall than in road traffic accidents, but the variation between countries in the extent of falls as a cause of death is very wide (Figure 1.7).

◆

COPD is the subject of another book in this series *Chronic Obstructive Pulmonary Disease: A Forgotten Killer* (Midgley, 2008).

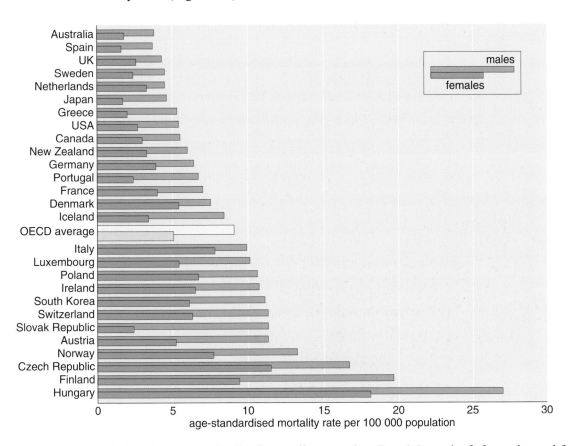

Figure 1.7 Variations in age-standardised mortality rates (see Box 1.1 overleaf) for males and females due to falls, per 100 000 population in OECD countries, in 2001 or 2002. (Source: OECD, 2005, Chart 1.16, p. 29)

The Organisation of Economic Cooperation and Development (OECD) is a confederation of 30 countries, committed to 'democratic government and market economics', which publishes reports and statistics on a range of economic and social issues, including health, science and innovation.

Box 1.1 (Explanation) Age-standardisation

Data on traumatic injury have to be 'age-standardised' before comparisons can be made between injury rates in countries where the proportion of the population in each age-group is different (e.g. developing countries tend to have more young people and fewer older people than are found in developed countries). Age-standardisation involves making a mathematical adjustment to the data from different countries which corrects for the distorting effects of differences in their age structures. It is particularly important to age-standardise data on injuries, because (as Table 1.1 illustrated) the distribution varies greatly between different age-groups, so the distortion would be significant if you compared data from an 'ageing' population such as the USA with that of a 'young' population such as Brazil.

1.2.3 Variations by gender

Globally, all categories of trauma result in many more deaths among males than females (Figures 1.7 and 1.8), with the exception of injuries caused by fires, which kill almost twice as many women as men in South-East Asian countries such as India, Bangladesh, Indonesia, Pakistan and Thailand, in Middle-Eastern states including Afghanistan, Egypt, Iraq and Iran, and in African Islamic countries such as Sudan, Morocco and Tunisia. One explanation for this pattern is that men in these cultures are not generally involved in domestic work, so women are much more likely than men to be killed in house fires, particularly those originating in cooking stoves. However, a proportion of these injuries and deaths are known to be intentional acts by family members who have set women alight as a punishment, or in dowry disputes, and attempted to disguise the fire as an accident (UNIFEM, 2002).

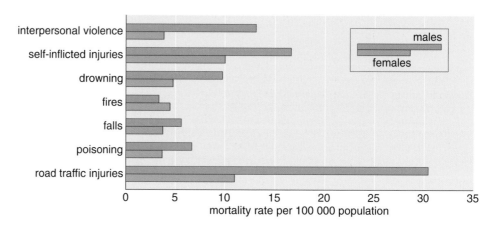

Figure 1.8   Global trauma-related mortality rates in 2000 for different causes of injury in males and females per 100 000 population in each sex. (Source: WHO, 2002, un-numbered bar chart, p. 14)

The mortality rates in Figure 1.8 are 'sex-standardised', i.e. male rates are expressed per 100 000 males in the population, and female rates are per 100 000 females.

Death rates in traffic accidents and from interpersonal violence are around three times higher among men than among women. The gap between male and female deaths from traumatic injuries is widest in Eastern Europe and Africa, where male rates are the highest in the world. Fatal accidental injuries sustained at work are about *fifteen* times higher in males than in females across the world (Concha-Barrientos et al., 2005).

1.3   Disability after surviving an injury

The most common international measure of **morbidity**, i.e. the burden of living with a disease, disorder or disability is the **disability adjusted life year** or **DALY** (pronounced 'daily': see Box 1.2). For every death from injury detailed in this chapter, several thousand people suffer a long-term physical or psychological disability and many thousands more are temporarily disabled. In the year 2000, the world's human inhabitants experienced over 182 million DALYs as a result of accidental or intentional injuries.

> **Box 1.2** (Explanation) Measuring the global burden of trauma-related disability
>
> DALYs combine an estimate of the number of years lived with a reduced quality of life due to a disease or disability (e.g. resulting from an injury), taking into account the severity of the condition, and the number of years of life lost if the person dies prematurely.

The variations reported earlier in the distribution of trauma-related *deaths* between different parts of the world, different age-groups and between males and females, also apply to the distribution of *non-fatal injuries*. A corollary of the gender bias in deaths reported above (Section 1.2.3) is the under-reporting of injury as a result of violence by men against their female partners. A review of more than 50 surveys in different parts of the world found that between 3% and 52% of women interviewed had been physically injured by their male partner in the previous year (Heise et al., 1999; reported in Watts and Zimmerman, 2002).

Survival from injury is often dependent on the level of subsequent care, and this applies not only to tissue repair (Chapter 5) but also recovery from psychological trauma (Chapter 6). People who suffer a life-threatening trauma in a low- or middle-income country are *six times* more likely to die from potentially treatable injuries than their counterparts in high-income countries (Mock et al., 2004). A global taskforce – the Essential Trauma Care Project – was set up in 2004 between the WHO and various international associations involved in trauma surgery and intensive care to try to address serious shortfalls in the use of equipment, the shortage of essential supplies and the inadequacy of staff training.

In the final part of this chapter, we focus on trauma arising from traffic accidents – the largest source of trauma-related injuries and deaths worldwide.

Traffic-related injuries in developing countries

In 2002, almost 1.2 million people died in traffic accidents and the number injured may have been as high as 50 million. Around 90% of these deaths and injuries occurred to people in developing countries, as Activity 1.1 illustrates.

Activity 1.1 'Road safety is no accident'

Allow 20 minutes

Now would be a good time to go to the DVD associated with this book and view the short film entitled 'Road safety is no accident', which was made by the WHO to promote World Health Day 2004. The film begins with the personal accounts of two people in different countries who were paralysed in road accidents, who speak about the effect on their lives, their psychological state and their families. It illustrates the importance of traffic-related trauma as a major public health issue, particularly in developing countries, using film from different locations and testimony from several heads of state in 2004 and the then Secretary General of the United Nations, Kofi Annan. If you are unable to do so now, continue studying the rest of the chapter and watch the video as soon as you can. While you are watching, make notes of the kinds of interventions that are proposed as ways to:

(a) prevent traffic accidents from occurring, and

(b) reduce the number of deaths and/or severity of injuries when accidents do occur.

As the WHO film illustrates, the types of road-users who are killed or injured in traffic accidents in developing countries are very different from those in high-income countries, where drivers of four-wheeled vehicles are the largest group (e.g. in the USA, over 60% of such deaths are to car drivers: Nantulya and Reich, 2002). In developing countries, at least three-quarters of traffic-related deaths and injuries are sustained by pedestrians, passengers and cyclists, including motor cyclists (Figure 1.9). There are at least twice as many bicycles in the world as there are cars, and in China over a third of all traffic-related deaths occur to bicyclists. Vignette 1.1 is a typical story about two boys on a motorcycle in Pakistan.

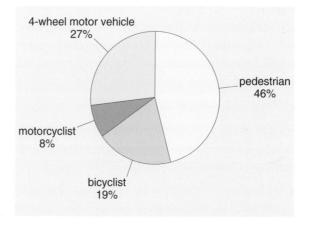

Figure 1.9 Percentage of deaths in traffic accidents suffered by different types of road users in rural Bangalore province, India, 1995–2002. (Source: Global Road Safety Partnership, 2004, un-numbered figure, p. 2)

Vignette 1.1   A motorcycle accident in Pakistan

Hassan, aged 16, was riding his motorcycle along a main road in the outskirts of Karachi with his six-year-old brother Wassim on the pillion, when he skidded on a patch of oil. The bike ran into the side of a bus travelling at speed on the wrong side of the road to overtake a slow-moving lorry. The bus swerved and crashed into a wall. This scenario is fairly typical of situations that lead to serious road traffic accidents, not only in Pakistan but throughout the developing world (Figure 1.10). The first national injury survey of traffic accidents in Pakistan reported that:

> Enforcement of existing traffic laws by police and other agencies in Pakistan is weak and in general confined to post-crash situations when damage has already been done.

(Ghaffar et al., 2004, p. 215)

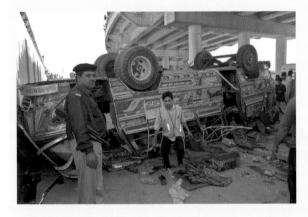

Figure 1.10   A crashed bus at the scene of an accident in Pakistan. (Source: Adnan Ali/AP/PA Photos)

Neither of the boys was wearing a crash helmet or protective clothing and they both had 'flip-flops' on their feet. Wassim was lucky and escaped with minor cuts and bruises, but Hassan's leg was trapped in the wreckage of his bike. His leg was broken, the leg muscles and skin were torn and crushed and he lost a considerable amount of blood. The boys were taken by a passing motorist to the Aga Khan University Hospital (a teaching hospital internationally recognised for providing quality healthcare, Figure 1.11)

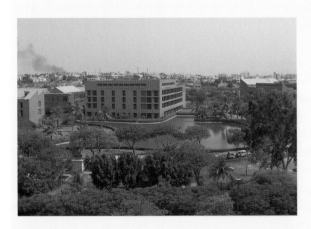

Figure 1.11   The Aga Khan University Hospital, Karachi, Pakistan. (Source: A. rehman Alvi/Flickr Photo Sharing)

for assessment and treatment. The hospital has a trauma resuscitation room, a diagnostic X-ray department, 24-hour availability of operating theatres and a multidisciplinary trauma team, serving the population of Karachi (about 12 million people).

Pre-hospital care for seriously injured people in Pakistan is reported to be either non-existent or of poor quality (Zafar et al., 2002). Only 6.5% of patients arrive by ambulance; the rest are brought in by citizens who happened to be on the scene, as in Hassan and Wassim's case.

The care that people receive immediately after an accident can be critical in determining the outcome of a traumatic injury. A concept of the 'golden hour' has been developed in western Accident and Emergency Departments, recognising that care during the first hour after an injury is the most important indicator of survival and subsequent recovery. Unfortunately, in most locations in developing countries the 'golden hour' concept cannot be fulfilled. Zafar and his colleagues (2002) studied 279 people treated at the emergency department of the Aga Khan University Hospital: the average time from injury to arrival in hospital of those who subsequently died from their injuries was 5.1 hours. Hassan and Wassim were lucky to get there in under an hour. You will find out what happened to Hassan in later chapters.

The concept of the 'golden hour' is explored further in DVD Activity 2.2a.

Finally, you should note that the cost of traffic-related trauma to national economies and individual families is colossal. We return to this point in more detail at the end of this book.

Summary of Chapter 1

1.1   Up to half a billion people are injured every year, 5 million of them fatally; injuries represent a major but neglected global health problem.

1.2   The distribution of injuries due to different causes varies between regions of the world, across different age-groups and between the sexes.

1.3   Around 90% of fatal injuries and trauma-related DALYs due to traffic accidents occur in low- and middle-income countries.

1.4   The greatest cause of fatal traumatic injury in children under 5 years is drowning; between 5 and 59 years it is traffic accidents, but poisoning, falls, fires, drowning, self-inflicted injuries, interpersonal violence and war are also important causes of death.

1.5   Male deaths from injuries outnumber female deaths for all causes except fires; a proportion of fire-related deaths among women in some developing countries are intentionally caused and violence by men against their female partners is under-reported.

Learning outcomes for Chapter 1

After studying this chapter and its associated activities, you should be able to:

LO 1.1   Define and use in context, or recognise definitions and applications of, each of the terms printed in **bold** in the text. (Question 1.1)

LO 1.2   Interpret data in graphs and tables as evidence that enables you to discuss the relative importance of traumatic injury due to different causes on a global level. (Question 1.1 and DVD Activity 1.1)

LO 1.3   Describe some of the factors that lead to increased risk of traumatic injury in certain populations and demographic groups. (Question 1.2)

LO 1.4   Use the sociological categories of age, gender and income group to illustrate how traffic-related traumatic injury is distributed in different populations. (Questions 1.1 and 1.2)

Self-assessment questions for Chapter 1

You also had the opportunity to demonstrate LO 1.2 by answering questions in Activity 1.1.

Question 1.1 (LOs 1.1, 1.2 and 1.4)

In less than 150 words, write a short description of the epidemiological data in Figure 1.12 in language that someone who has not studied this chapter or seen the diagram could understand. In your description, you should compare male and female deaths at different ages, by referring to approximate numbers of deaths as shown in Figure 1.12.

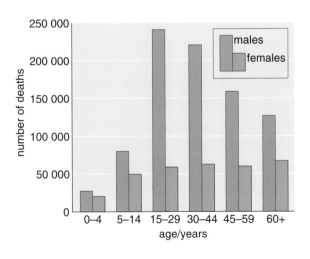

Figure 1.12 Bar chart showing the distribution of worldwide deaths from traffic-related injuries in 2002, by sex and age group. (Source: data from Peden et al., 2004, Figure 2.8, p. 45)

Question 1.2 (LOs 1.3 and 1.4)

Why do you think the incidence of death and injury from road crashes is rising in low- and middle-income countries such as India and Pakistan, yet falling in high-income countries where there are many more motor vehicles per head of population?

CHAPTER 2

INITIAL RESPONSE TO SERIOUS INJURY

2.1   Acute life-threatening conditions

Traumatic injuries take many forms, from road accidents and falls to gunshot wounds and burns. The ability of a trauma patient to recover will depend on many factors such as the severity of the injury, the availability of care and the person's age and health. Before looking in detail at the nature of damage to certain body tissues, and the mechanisms that enable them to repair, it is important that you gain an understanding of the life-threatening aspects of traumatic injuries.

In the first instance, the survival of a person who has experienced a serious traumatic injury will depend on the extent of damage that occurs to essential body systems. If one of these systems is severely impaired, then the person is likely to die within minutes of an injury. The survival of a person with damage to their essential body systems can depend entirely on the immediate care provided. Many lives have been saved through rapid provision of basic life support by the first people to reach the scene. The concept of a 'golden hour' (introduced in Section 1.3) has been widely adopted by healthcare workers involved in emergency care. This refers to the idea that following serious trauma there is a limited length of time a person can survive without specialist *surgical* treatment. The golden hour is the 60 minutes following injury and it is generally accepted that a person's chance of survival is greatest if they receive surgery before the hour has elapsed.

2.1.1   Damage to the cardiovascular system

In order to sustain life, the cells of the body need an adequate supply of oxygen. This comes from the air breathed into the lungs and is distributed around the body by blood circulation. The circuit involving the heart and the blood vessels is known as the **cardiovascular system** (*cardio-* refers to the heart and *vascular* refers to the blood vessels). Any disruption to this system will mean that body cells are deprived of oxygen and will cease to function. In trauma, disruption might be in the form of damage to the pump that moves the blood around (the heart) or damage to the blood vessels resulting in a loss of blood and a decrease in blood pressure (Section 2.2).

The flow of blood (and therefore oxygen) around the body is carefully controlled to ensure an adequate supply to meet tissue requirements. During rest, heart rate (the number of beats per minute) and breathing slow to a rate that will provide sufficient oxygen to support the continuous energy-requiring processes in the body. During exercise, the muscles use oxygen at a faster rate than at rest, so the heart rate increases along with the breathing rate in order to meet this extra demand. If blood circulation is impaired by trauma, the resulting lack of oxygen to the brain will rapidly result in a loss of consciousness as the brain cells can no longer perform their energy-requiring functions.

2.1.2   Disruption to the airway, breathing and circulation

Entry of air to the lungs depends on the presence of an open airway through the mouth or nose and down the trachea (windpipe) to the lungs

(Figure 2.1). If this airway becomes blocked either through direct injury or because of an obstruction (commonly the casualty's own blood or vomit), then no air reaches the lungs and consequently no oxygen can diffuse into the blood. If a person becomes unconscious through injury or illness, then their airway can become blocked by the back of their tongue. Emergency intervention to clear the airway, perhaps by removing an obstruction or inserting a tube (or even just tilting the head back to bring the tongue forward), is a priority.

Diffusion is the movement of molecules from regions of high concentration into regions of lower concentration.

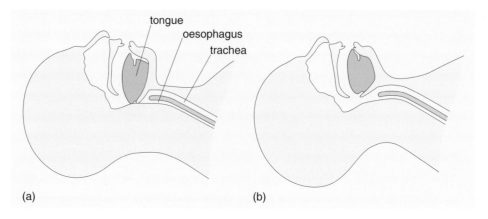

Figure 2.1 Diagram of a person's airway: (a) blocked by their tongue and (b) cleared by tilting the head and lifting the chin.

Techniques such as these can save lives, but in order to be effective and not cause further harm, proper training is necessary.

If the airway is clear but the person is not breathing, then the lungs can be ventilated artificially by blowing air in through the mouth using a bag valve mask (Figure 2.2) or using the exhaled breath of another person. This latter method is possible because not all of the oxygen in a single breath diffuses into the blood in the lungs, so exhaled air (in this case, exhaled by the aid-giver) still contains sufficient oxygen to sustain life.

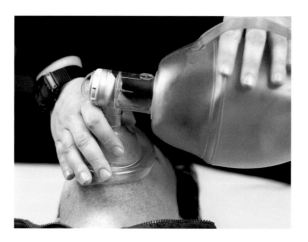

Figure 2.2 A bag valve mask being used to ventilate a person's lungs. (Source: Leonid Smirnov/ iStockphoto)

Getting oxygen into the lungs is not the end of the story; the oxygen diffuses into the blood in the pulmonary capillaries but then must be delivered to the tissues by the circulation of the blood. This takes place via the cardiovascular system: a network of fluid-filled pipes (blood vessels) with a central pump (the heart) which is responsible for moving the blood around. This movement is possible because this is a closed system – as the heart squeezes more blood into the network in one place (increasing the pressure), blood moves around all of the other parts of the system. The **arteries** are the vessels that carry the blood away from the heart and they have thick muscular walls to support this pressurised flow (Figure 2.3).

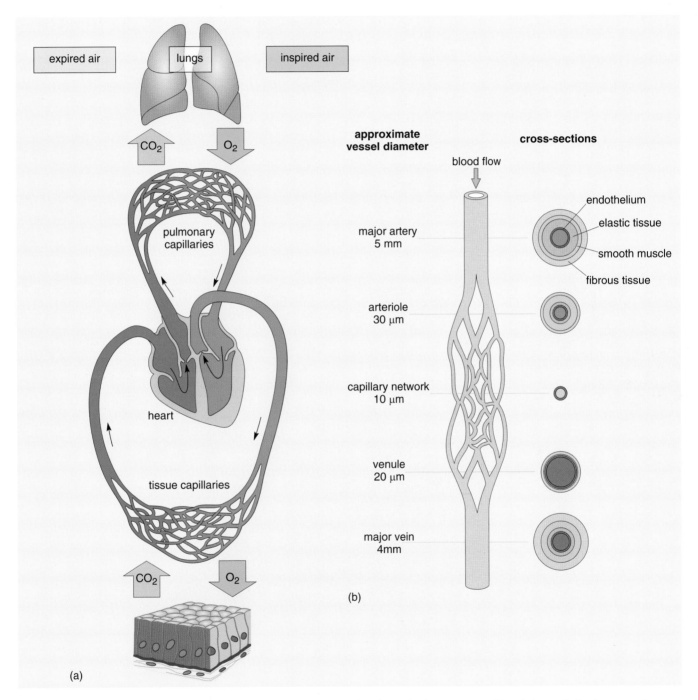

Figure 2.3 (a) Summary of the cardiovascular system showing how the heart pumps blood through the lungs and through the other tissues of the body. (b) Approximate vessel diameter and cross-sections through the different types of blood vessel. Arteries and arterioles carry pressurised blood away from the heart, whereas veins and venules do not carry blood under high pressure. These differences in function are reflected in the structure of the walls of the vessels; in particular note the thick layers of elastic tissue and smooth muscle in the walls of the arteriole compared with the venule.

The arteries lead via smaller arteries, known as arterioles, into much smaller **capillaries**, which are thin-walled vessels that carry the blood through the tissues where the oxygen is used. Then the deoxygenated blood (blood depleted in oxygen) flows back to the heart via the venules and **veins** (blood in the veins is not highly pressurised like that in the arteries so these vessels have thinner walls; Activity 2.1 will explain how blood moves through the veins). Any damage to the body that results in a substantial loss of blood will impair this system – blood loss will reduce blood pressure and the pumping of the heart will no longer provide an adequate blood flow to supply sufficient oxygen to the tissues.

Activity 2.1 Demonstrating venous return

Allow about 10 minutes

Blood in the veins is not as highly pressurised as the blood in the arteries, so how does it return from the tissues to the heart at a sufficient rate to enable it to be pumped through the lungs to collect oxygen and then back through the heart and into the arteries?

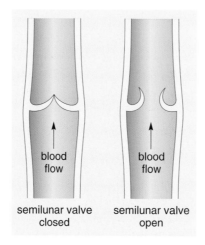

blood flow

blood flow

semilunar valve closed

semilunar valve open

Figure 2.4 Valves inside the veins ensure blood flows in one direction. The valves are known as semi-lunar because of their 'half moon' shape.

The flow of blood back to the heart in the veins is known as **venous return** and is achieved by the presence of valves in the veins which only allow blood to flow in one direction, that is, *towards* the heart (Figure 2.4). These valves mean that whenever a vein is squashed slightly due to the contraction of nearby muscles during normal movement, the blood within it moves towards the heart – not away from it. Other factors influence venous return including gravity – you might like to try these simple experiments to illustrate the effect of gravity and body movements on venous return (note that these are fun to try but do not always work clearly, so don't worry if you don't see an effect).

◆ In either a sitting or standing position, hold one arm straight up in the air, keeping your hand above your head, whilst you let the other arm relax hanging by your side. Keep this position for about 30 seconds, then hold both hands next to each other in front of you and compare them. Do you see any differences?

◆ The hand that was held up should be paler in colour than the one that was hanging by your side. This is because during the 30 seconds of the experiment, more blood drained out of the raised hand than the lowered one since the blood flow in the veins in the raised arm was assisted by gravity pulling it back down your arm.

Further illustration of venous return can be seen with the following experiment, which you can try after the colour in both hands has returned to normal.

◆ Let *both* hands hang by your sides this time, but for 30 seconds constantly clench and release one hand whilst keeping the other one still. When you immediately hold both hands out in front of you after the 30 seconds, do you see any differences?

◆ The hand that was clenching should be paler in colour than the one that was kept still. This is a demonstration of the effect of muscle contraction on venous return – in the moving forearm and hand, the veins were being squeezed far more than in the other forearm and hand, so more blood was moved along the veins towards the heart. It is interesting to note that, in this case, this blood was being moved *against* gravity. Most of the time, the blood in the veins in the limbs has to flow uphill against gravity (as opposed to the blood in the veins of the head, which flows downhill most of the time).

2.2 Blood pressure measurement and blood loss

Blood pressure is frequently discussed in the context of health and disease, and people are often referred to as having 'high blood pressure', which is associated with increased risk of heart disease and strokes. If *high* blood pressure is risky, and *low* blood pressure after blood loss can starve tissues of oxygen, then an understanding of exactly what the measurement of blood pressure refers to is clearly important.

Pressure in this case is a measure of how hard the blood is pushing on the walls of the arteries. The units used traditionally for measuring pressure in blood are 'millimetres of mercury' (abbreviated to mmHg, where mm stands for millimetres and Hg is the chemical symbol for mercury, a metal that is liquid at room temperature). These units are derived from one of the ways that pressure can be measured: if mercury is contained in a U-tube (an instrument called a *manometer*, Figure 2.5), the height to which the mercury column is pushed up one arm of the U-tube is directly related to the pressure applied to the other end. Instruments for measuring blood pressure (*sphygmomanometers*; 'sfig–mo')

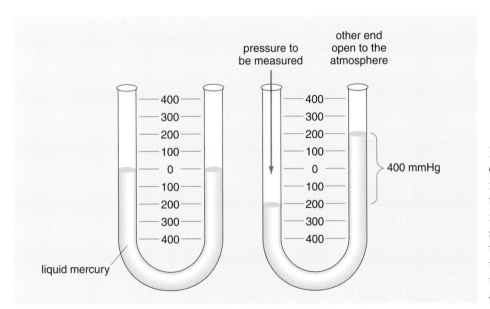

Figure 2.5 Schematic diagram of a manometer. The difference in air pressure on either side of the column of liquid mercury in the tube can be read from the scale as the difference between the heights of the two sides of the column. In this diagram the pressure difference is 400 mmHg.

that contain mercury have now largely been replaced by electronic devices, but mmHg remains the accepted unit for blood pressure.

Measurement of blood pressure

The pressure of blood pressing on the walls of the arteries increases each time the heart pumps more blood into the arterial system. Between each contraction of the heart, the pressure in the arteries decreases and this alternating increase and decrease in pressure causes the 'pulse' that can be felt in the arteries. Blood pressure measurements are expressed as two different numbers: the **systolic** (pronounced 'sis-tollic') pressure is the high pressure in the arteries that occurs *during* heart contraction and is typically around 120 mmHg in healthy adults. The **diastolic** (dye-a-stollic) pressure is the lower pressure in the arteries that occurs *between* heart contractions and is typically around 80 mmHg in healthy adults. Blood pressure is expressed as 'systolic/diastolic' or 'systolic over diastolic', for example '120 over 80 mmHg'. Some typical blood pressure values are listed in Table 2.1.

Table 2.1 Blood pressure values for normal, low (hypotension) and high (hypertension) states. Stage 1 hypertension is an early form of high blood pressure that may require treatment to avoid progression to stage 2 hypertension, which is a serious form of high blood pressure requiring immediate treatment. (Adapted from Seventh report of the Joint National Committee on Prevention, Detection, Evaluation, and Treatment of High Blood Pressure, NIH Publication No. 03-5233, May 2003)

Category	Systolic/mmHg	Diastolic/mmHg
hypotension	less than 90	less than 60
normal	90–120	60–80
stage 1 hypertension	140–159	90–99
stage 2 hypertension	160 or higher	100 or higher

The measurement of blood pressure can be carried out using a cuff around the arm, which can be inflated with air in order to squash the arteries enough to stop blood flow (Figure 2.6). As the cuff is gradually deflated, blood flow is restored and the pressure in the cuff is monitored. Initially, the cuff pressure is higher than systolic pressure so no blood flows. At the point when cuff pressure is reduced to the same level as systolic pressure, blood starts to squirt through the squashed arteries in a turbulent manner (turbulence is a disruption of fluid flow, in this case caused by the artificial narrowing of the arteries by the cuff). This moment can be detected by listening to the area with a stethoscope – the pressure of the cuff (displayed on the gauge of the sphygmomanometer) equals systolic pressure at this point and becomes the first of the two blood pressure readings. The second reading (diastolic) is obtained at the moment when turbulence stops – this is the point at which the cuff pressure no longer interferes with blood flow through the arteries.

Blood pressure is controlled by both the rate and size of heart contractions (cardiac output) and the constriction and dilation of blood vessels (peripheral resistance). Signals from the nervous system maintain an effective circulation during different activities (changes in oxygen demand from organs, changes in posture, etc.).

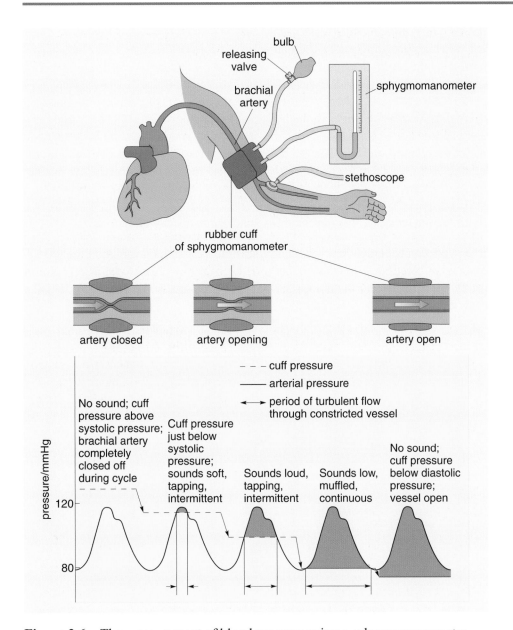

Figure 2.6 The measurement of blood pressure using a sphygmomanometer. The cuff around the arm is inflated using the bulb and the pressure in the cuff is monitored with the gauge on the sphygmomanometer. Initially the cuff pressure is sufficiently high to close the artery completely, then the cuff pressure is gradually reduced until the artery is fully open. The dashed line on the graph shows the pressure in the cuff being reduced in stages – the red area indicates the amount of blood that can flow through the artery at each stage. The solid line shows the rise and fall in arterial pressure that occurs with each contraction of the heart and the descriptions explain what can be heard through the stethoscope at each stage. (Source: van Wynsberghe et al., 1995)

Most adults can afford to lose 10% of their blood volume without experiencing any problems (a typical adult male has about 5 litres of blood so 10% is about 500 ml, the volume normally donated with no ill effects by a blood donor). If more blood is lost (about 20%) through serious bleeding following trauma, then there is an initial

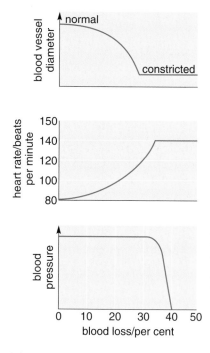

Figure 2.7 Changes in blood vessel dilation, heart rate and blood pressure with increasing blood loss. (Source: Barraclough, 2006)

decrease in systolic blood pressure, which triggers a nervous system response. This response acts to counteract the drop in blood pressure by increasing heart rate and narrowing the capillaries that carry blood to the skin (Figure 2.7 and Table 2.2). This condition is called **hypovolaemic shock** (*hypo-* means low and *volaemic* (voll-eemic) refers to blood volume). Raised heart rate and pale cold skin are the classic symptoms. Increasing heart rate and reducing the amount of blood passing through less vital organs (e.g. the skin) is the body's attempt to maintain blood pressure and therefore a steady supply of oxygen to the tissues. However, when large volumes of blood are lost, then the heart cannot beat any faster and the blood vessels are unable to constrict any further, so these changes are insufficient to maintain blood flow to the brain and other vital organs, leading to confusion and unconsciousness. If lost fluids are not replaced, then severe shock will lead to death within minutes.

It is important to remember that blood loss following trauma can be in the form of *internal* bleeding – this means that blood is being lost from a damaged vein or artery but is not escaping through the skin and instead is accumulating within a body cavity.

◆ Apart from a reduction in blood volume caused by blood loss, what else could lead to an inadequate supply of blood to the tissues (shock)?

◆ Damage to the heart muscle (e.g. through trauma or a heart attack) could also cause shock, because the transport of blood to the tissues would be impaired if the heart failed to pump effectively.

Table 2.2 The effects of different volumes of blood loss on a person's consciousness, skin colour and feel, pulse rate and breathing rate. (Adapted from Barraclough, 2006). Values shown for pulse and breathing rates are *typical* values for an adult at rest following blood loss; in reality these might vary considerably with blood loss following trauma (e.g. as a result of pain or anxiety).

Blood loss:	10%	20%	30%	40% +
consciousness	normal	may feel dizzy	lowered consciousness level; restless, anxious	unresponsive
skin	normal	pale	cyanosis (pale grey tinges to the lips and skin), cold and clammy	severe cyanosis, cold and clammy
pulse	normal (60–80 per min)	slightly raised (80–100 per min)	rapid (over 100 per min), hard to detect	undetectable
breathing	normal (12–20 per min)	slightly raised (20–30 per min)	rapid (over 30 per min)	deep sighing breaths

2.3 Damage to the nervous system

In addition to direct damage to the airway, lungs or circulation, damage to those parts of the nervous system that control heart contraction and breathing can be life-threatening. This damage could be caused directly to the nervous system, or may be a result of a reduction in the supply of oxygenated blood which would starve the brain cells of the oxygen they need in order to function and survive.

Nervous system damage can be assessed following traumatic injury by the level of response that a patient shows to various stimuli. One system for assessing this level of response is the Glasgow Coma Scale (GCS) shown in Table 2.3, which measures the extent to which a patient can respond to spoken instructions and painful skin stimuli. The response is measured by looking at the eye movements, limb movements, and listening to the verbal responses to questions.

Table 2.3 The Glasgow Coma Scale. Because individual elements as well as an overall responsiveness value are important, the score is expressed in the form (for example) 'GCS 12 = E4 M5 V3 at 09:30' where 12 is the sum of the three response values E, M and V assessed at time 09:30.

Eye response	Movement	Verbal response
4 – spontaneous	6 – obeys commands	5 – totally alert
3 – to speech	5 – points to pain	4 – seems confused
2 – to pain	4 – withdraws from pain	3 – inappropriate words
1 – none	3 – bends limbs to pain	2 – utters sounds
	2 – stretches limbs to pain	1 – none
	1 – none	

◆ Why do you think it is useful to be able to *quantify* a person's level of response in this manner?

◆ Using a quantitative approach gives medical staff a rapid way of communicating and recording a person's level of response, and repeated assessment done in the same way enables any subsequent improvement or deterioration to be easily identified.

Now would be a good time to go to the DVD associated with this book and work through Activity 2.2, which is based around the training that paramedics in the UK receive in order to provide emergency care at the scene of a traumatic injury.

Activity 2.2a   Care at the scene of an injury

Activity 2.2b   Simulating responses to trauma

Allow about 1 hour

The video for Activity 2.2a shows trainees and instructors responding to a simulated road-traffic collision in which they assess and stabilise a casualty, who is played by an actor, then remove him from the car into an ambulance. You will hear the paramedics talking about the 'golden hour' and some of the treatments a patient can receive before they reach hospital, including pain control (Box 2.1).

In Activity 2.2b, a video sequence introduces a computerised dummy used in the training of ambulance staff. This is followed by an interactive exercise that simulates some of the responses a person would exhibit following injury and enables you to choose what intervention to make to prevent their condition from deteriorating.

Pain is the subject of another book in this series (Toates, 2007).

Box 2.1 (Explanation) Pain

Pain is something that people tend to associate with tissue damage, but as you heard in Activity 2.2, the most serious tissue damage is not necessarily accompanied by the greatest pain. This is because pain depends upon various factors, only one of which is the extent of any tissue damage. It depends also on the individual circumstances of that person at that moment in time (e.g. relief following rescue or fear of the future). Because of this, pain relief in the form of drugs is given following an assessment of the needs of the individual in terms of the amount of pain that they report feeling. It can be difficult to form a reliable prediction of the amount of pain likely to result from a particular injury.

Once the initial life-threatening factors following traumatic injury have been identified, assessed and stabilised, the extent of damage to tissues and organs within the body can be investigated. Some of these procedures will be discussed in the next chapter. However, in addition to the physical damage caused by a traumatic injury, there are often psychological effects which are likely to vary between people and situations. Occasionally the psychological effects of receiving or witnessing a traumatic injury can persist long after the physical damage has healed. This disorder, known as *post-traumatic stress disorder*, will be described in Chapter 6.

Summary of Chapter 2

2.1   The cardiovascular system circulates oxygen from the lungs to the cells and vital organs in the body. Initial life-threatening effects of traumatic injury are those that disrupt this system, by interfering with the airway, breathing or circulation.

2.2   Blood is pumped around the body through the arteries under pressure. Systolic and diastolic blood pressure readings give an indication of how well the cardiovascular system is functioning.

2.3   After passing through the tissues in small capillaries, blood returns to the heart in the veins, moved along by compression of the veins due to contraction of nearby muscles. The presence of one-way valves means the blood in veins only moves towards the heart.

2.4   Blood loss can result in hypovolaemic shock, the seriousness of which increases with the volume of blood lost. The body responds to hypovolaemic shock by constricting blood vessels and increasing heart rate in an attempt to maintain blood pressure.

2.5   If the brain is starved of oxygen, then the level of consciousness can be impaired. This can range from reduced responses to stimuli, to life-threatening nervous system damage.

Learning outcomes for Chapter 2

After studying this chapter and its associated activities, you should be able to:

LO 2.1   Define and use in context, or recognise definitions and applications of, each of the terms printed in **bold** in the text. (Question 2.1)

LO 2.2   Describe the importance of basic life-support concepts in the context of traumatic injury (airway, breathing, circulation, bleeding and consciousness). (Question 2.2 and DVD Activity 2.2)

LO 2.3   Describe how blood pressure is generated in the cardiovascular system and demonstrate an understanding of how and why it is measured, and what constitute typical (systolic/diastolic) values and acceptable limits. Associate changes in measured blood pressure, heart rate and breathing with events following trauma (blood loss, shock). (Questions 2.2, 2.3 and 2.4, Activity 2.1 and DVD Activity 2.2)

LO 2.4   Describe the differences between arteries and veins in terms of their overall structure and the means by which blood moves through each (arterial pressure and venous return). (Questions 2.1 and 2.4 and Activity 2.1)

Self-assessment questions for Chapter 2

You also had the opportunity to demonstrate LOs 2.2 and 2.3 by completing DVD Activity 2.2.

Question 2.1 (LOs 2.1 and 2.4)

Briefly describe how the blood moves through different parts of the cardiovascular system, referring to the blood vessels involved and any structural features associated with blood movement.

Question 2.2 (LOs 2.2 and 2.3)

Explain the sequence of events that you would predict to occur in a person who was bleeding uncontrollably from a damaged artery.

Question 2.3 (LO 2.3)

What effect on blood pressure would you expect to see if the blood vessels in a person's skin constricted? How else could this effect on blood pressure be achieved?

Question 2.4 (LOs 2.3 and 2.4)

Soldiers on parade who need to stand very still for long periods of time are trained to clench and release their calf muscles gently to prevent fainting (fainting occurs when the body detects reduced blood flow to the brain). Can you suggest how this technique might work?

CHAPTER 3

UNDERSTANDING THE STRUCTURE OF TISSUES

3.1 Introduction

This chapter will consider the structure of tissues that may be damaged during traumatic injury. It will focus on the leg as an example of a region of the body that is frequently damaged. We return for a moment to the scene of the accident in Pakistan (Vignette 3.1).

Vignette 3.1 Hassan's initial treatment

Hassan sustained a serious injury to his leg, which involved damage to many different tissues. At the scene of the accident, there were no paramedics, but there were members of the public who knew to protect themselves and the casualties from danger (mainly by directing traffic away from the scene) and to check Hassan and Wassim for any initial life-threatening conditions (i.e. checking for clear airway, breathing and circulation). Hassan's blood loss was the primary concern and attempts were made to minimise his bleeding by applying pressure to the open wounds on his leg while he was taken as swiftly as possible to the hospital. The damage to the tissues in Hassan's leg meant that he was in a lot of pain during this short journey, made worse by the application of pressure to stop the bleeding, and the rough movements of the car as it raced through the streets. On arrival at hospital, the medical staff rapidly assessed Hassan's condition, checking his airway, breathing and circulation again and measuring his heart rate, blood pressure and level of consciousness. The bleeding had been stopped effectively by the pressure applied at the scene and his level of consciousness was good (this was apparent by his cries of pain whenever anyone touched his injured leg). The medical staff were able to relieve Hassan's pain by giving him morphine; then a proper examination of Hassan's injured leg was possible. When Hassan later talked about what he remembered, he was surprised that he couldn't recall any initial pain at the scene, although he remembered the accident very clearly, but during the journey to the hospital the pain was excruciating and only abated when the doctors gave pain-relief drugs.

The detailed examination of Hassan's leg revealed that he had sustained damage mainly to the thigh. The doctors explained that he would need an operation to realign the broken bone and that there would be a long period of convalescence before he would be able to walk again.

3.2 Tissue structure

3.2.1 What is a tissue?

Before embarking on a detailed investigation of the structure of the leg and how it relates to function, it is worth pausing to think about the term 'tissue'.

A **tissue** is broadly defined as the substance and structure of part of the body. More specifically, in biology it is used to refer to a collection of similar cells that are grouped together in an organised manner to fulfil a particular function. Structure and function are intimately linked in the human body.

People are multicellular organisms, so different types of cells and other substances connect together to form tissues that perform specific functions in the body. There are several types of tissue. *Muscle tissues* allow movement and *nerve tissues* provide communication and control of body functions. *Epithelial tissues* are layers of cells that form either a barrier (e.g. the skin) or an interface across which substances are absorbed or secreted (e.g. the lining of the lungs or the gut). Finally, *connective tissues* support and connect cells and structures in the body, e.g. the bones, and the tendons which connect bones and muscles together.

◆ Make a list of the main tissues you think you would find in a leg.

◆ Your answer may have included bones, muscles, skin, blood vessels, ligaments, tendons, nerves, cartilage and fat.

This section will focus on bones, muscles, tendons, nerves, skin and blood vessels, outlining their structure and function and how they interact with each other under normal conditions. The final part of this chapter will discuss how damage can occur; then Chapters 4 and 5 will discuss how this damage can be controlled and repaired. There is an accompanying DVD activity which gives a more visual description, in particular providing information on how the different tissues are arranged around each other in the leg. We recommend that you work through Chapter 3, to gain some understanding of each of the main tissues independently, then study DVD Activity 3.1 to build up an integrated view of leg anatomy. By the end of Chapter 3, you should have an understanding of the variety of structures that make up a limb and how they interact as the limb functions.

'Anatomy' refers to the structure and arrangement of the different parts of the body, as determined by dismantling or dissecting it.

3.2.2 Overview of the musculoskeletal system and its functions

The limbs form part of the **musculoskeletal system**. This is the term used to refer to the system of muscles and bones and their various *joints* and linkages which facilitate support and movement. The *bones* provide a stiff strong framework which supports the other structures in the body. Here we are concerned with the bones in the limbs, which are primarily involved in movement, but other bony structures such as the skull and the ribs have the role of protecting softer tissues such as the brain and the internal organs of the chest. Movement of bones is achieved by contraction of *muscles* which are attached to the bones via strong rope-like structures called *tendons*.

The tissues are supplied with oxygen and nutrients via the blood, which travels throughout all of the tissues in *blood vessels*, carried from the heart to the limbs via arteries, then into the tissues via capillaries, then back to the heart in the veins (Chapter 2). Movement is controlled by signals from the brain; sensations such as pressure, pain and temperature are transmitted back to the brain, via the *nerves*. The limbs are protected by the *skin* which forms a barrier between the tissues and the outside world.

Before looking in more depth at the cells and other components that enable these tissues to perform their functions, the manner in which limb movement operates at a system level will be considered.

Because muscles cannot push, they can only pull, they generally work in pairs to achieve controlled limb movement. This is known as *antagonism* and the muscles are referred to as being *antagonistic pairs* (Figure 3.1). Bones meet at joints, and muscles that move bones closer together (known as *flexion*, e.g. bending the arm at the elbow or bending the leg at the knee) are *flexors*, whilst those that move bones further apart (known as *extension*, e.g. straightening the arm or leg) are *extensors*.

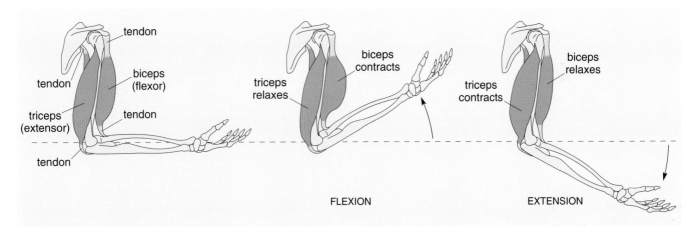

Figure 3.1 Diagram of arm movement showing flexors and extensors working in antagonistic pairs.

Muscles pull bones by contraction – when a muscle contracts it get shorter and thicker (there is no change in volume, just a change in shape). This shortening pulls on the tendon, which transfers the movement of the contraction to the bone, which moves. At the same time, the other muscle in the antagonistic pair must relax, to enable the bone to move. Movement within the musculoskeletal system is based on these principles, and the various bones work as **levers**. Levers are explained in Box 3.1 overleaf – they are simple devices that move in response to forces. **Force** is a term used to explain the size and direction of a push or pull.

Box 3.1 (Explanation) Archimedes and the principle of the lever

◇ Imagine a child and an adult on a see-saw. How could the much heavier adult position themselves to balance the weight of the light child?

◆ If the adult sat closer to the pivot point, then the see-saw would balance.

However, the adult would then not move up and down as much as the child. That is the essence of a lever – a small force can balance a large one, but as the lever moves the *smaller* force travels through a *larger* distance. The interplay between force and distance means that levers can be used in two roles. Often you want to use a modest force (your own strength perhaps) to move something very heavy. Using a lever helps. If the heavy item is near the **fulcrum** (the pivot point) it can easily be moved, but not very far (Figure 3.2).

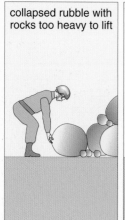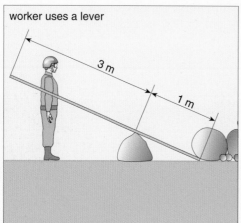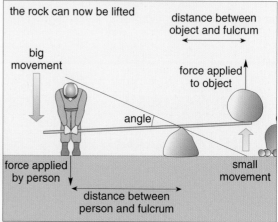

Figure 3.2 A rescue worker uses a lever to lift a heavy rock.

Alternatively, the lever can be used the other way round. In this case, a large force is used to move the short end of the lever over a relatively small distance, but the long end of the lever moves over a much greater distance.

The Greek mathematician Archimedes, who lived in the third century BC, is credited with first describing the principle of the lever by considering the forces applied at each end of the lever, and relating them to their distance from the fulcrum. His equation (below) shows how forces and distances in levers are related:

force applied to object × distance between object and fulcrum =
force applied by person × distance between person and fulcrum

Figure 3.2 shows that for a 4 m lever, with a fulcrum at 1 m from the end, the rescue worker is able to apply a force equivalent to three times his strength to the heavy rock.

force applied to object (N) × 1 m = person's strength (N) × 3 m

◆ ─────────────────

The unit of force is the newton (N).

As shown in Figure 3.2, levers consist of three important points: the position where the force is applied (i.e. the rescue worker), the fulcrum and the point where the lever moves the load (i.e. the rock). There are three types of lever found in the human body, each type being distinguished by the relative positions of these three points. In the body, the applied force (from muscle contraction) acts at the point where the tendon is connected to the bone. The fulcrum is the joint around which the lever (bone) moves, and the load is the force that resists the movement (for example, the object being lifted) (Figure 3.3).

 If you are studying this book as part of an Open University course, this would be a good point to try Activity C1 described in the *Companion*.

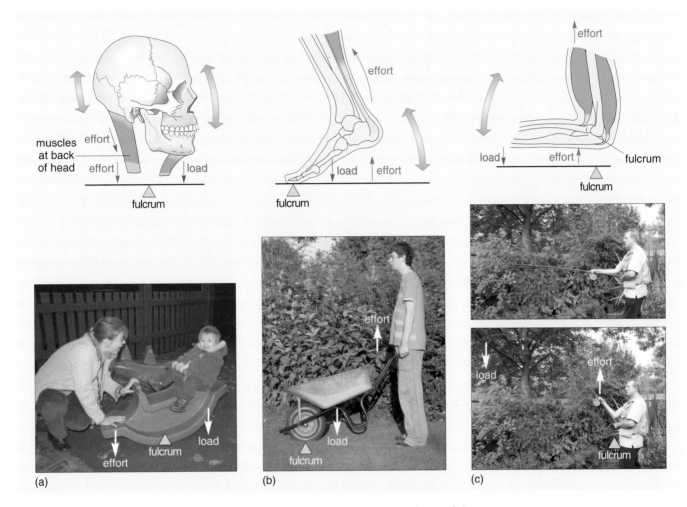

Figure 3.3 Levers fall into three 'classes' based on the relative positions of the applied force (effort), the fulcrum and the load being moved. (a) Class 1 levers have the fulcrum between the effort and the load as in a see-saw; an example in the body is nodding the head. (Source: Vicky Taylor) (b) Class 2 levers have the load between the effort and the fulcrum as in a wheelbarrow; an example in the body is the calf muscle lifting the leg. (c) Class 3 levers have the effort between the fulcrum and the load, like the man in the picture who uses his left hand as the fulcrum and lifts the far end of the rod (load) using his right hand (effort). An example of a class 3 lever in the body is the forearm being raised (load) by the biceps attached to the bone via a tendon (effort) at a point between the hand and the elbow (fulcrum).

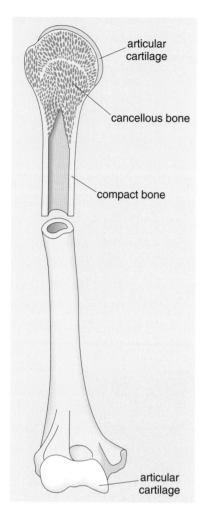

Figure 3.4 Diagram of a typical long bone in the leg.

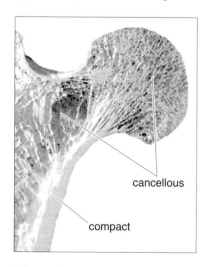

Figure 3.5 Longitudinal section through part of the head and neck of a femur showing cancellous and compact bone. (Source: Kerr, 1999)

3.3 The structures of individual tissues

When one considers tissues as diverse as bones, skin, nerves, etc. it is not obvious that they are, in fact, built in a very similar manner to each other, and from fairly similar materials. The general structure of all tissues is that cells are carefully arranged within an **extracellular matrix**, which holds them in place and in many cases forms the bulk material of the tissue. The term 'extracellular' refers to the fact that this material is *outside* the cells, whilst 'matrix' indicates that this is a substance in which the cells are embedded. Extracellular matrix is mainly made from proteins, which are large molecules with complex structures that enable them to fulfil a range of biological functions. You will probably have heard of other types of protein: for example, those that function as enzymes to catalyse biological reactions (e.g. alcohol dehydrogenase in the liver), or cell surface receptors to which signalling molecules specifically bind (e.g. neurotransmitter receptors at synapses between neurons in the nervous system), or blood proteins that carry oxygen (e.g. haemoglobin in red blood cells).

Proteins in the extracellular matrix tend to be shaped appropriately to fulfil the specific function of the tissue. For example, they form strong fibres in bone but are more flexible in skin allowing it to stretch. In all cases, the extracellular matrix proteins are *made* by cells, can be *modified* by cells, and provide the *structural properties* of the tissue (i.e. its strength and flexibility). This section looks at individual tissues in detail, starting with bone, whose remarkable structure makes it the central component of the musculoskeletal system.

3.3.1 Bones

It is a common misconception that hard parts of bones are predominantly made from dead material. In fact, they are riddled with living cells, complete with a blood supply and nerves. A cross-sectional view of a typical bone is shown in Figure 3.4.

◆ Figure 3.4 shows a 'long bone' such as those found in the arms and legs. Other types of bone include 'short', 'irregular' and 'flat' bones. Can you think of where in the human skeleton you might find an example of each of these other types?

◆ Short bones are found in the wrists and ankles, irregular bones include the vertebrae in the spine, and flat bones include the scapula (shoulder blade) and most skull bones.

The long bone in Figure 3.4 shows the typical structure: a long shaft which is wider at the ends where it meets other bones at the joints. There are two distinct types of bone tissue which can be seen in Figure 3.4: along the length of the shaft and all around the ends is **compact** (sometimes called *cortical*) bone, which is dense and forms a hollow cylinder; within this is less dense **cancellous** (can-sell-us) bone, which has a honeycomb appearance and fills the widened areas inside the ends of the bone. Figure 3.5 is a photograph of the inside of the end of a femur (the long bone in the upper part of the leg) showing the two types of bone.

Compact bone looks very dense in Figure 3.5, but using a microscope to look at it closely reveals that there are canals running through it containing fluid, cells and blood and lymph vessels (Figure 3.6). This type of bone is very strong, and thicker layers of compact bone are found in the parts of bones that need to withstand the largest forces. Cancellous bone fills the spaces within the ends of the bones and is considerably less dense but is arranged such that the numerous struts or *trabeculae* (trab-eck-you-lee) add extra strength to these regions (Figure 3.7).

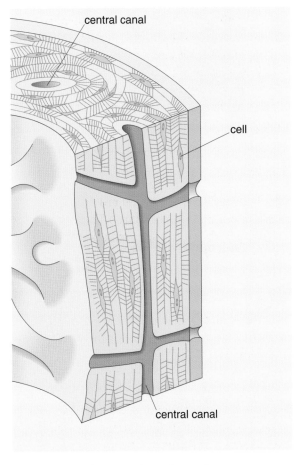

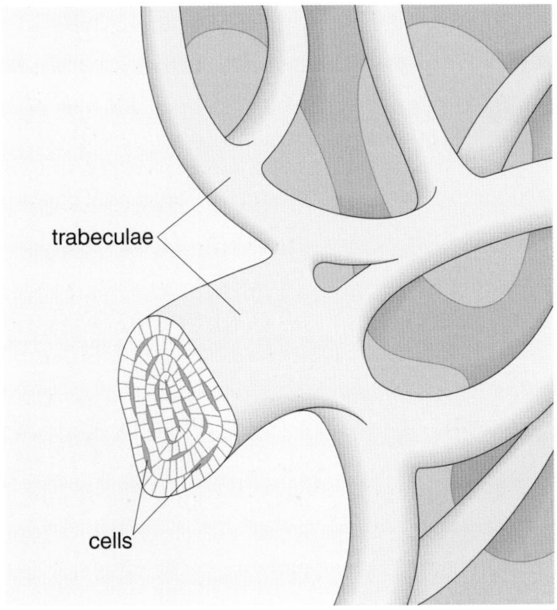

Figure 3.7 Cancellous bone is less dense than compact bone and contains trabeculae (struts) that give it strength.

Figure 3.6 Compact bone has a dense structure but contains cells and numerous canals in which blood vessels, lymph vessels and nerves are found.

◆ Can you suggest why bones are not entirely composed of dense compact bone?

◆ Compact bone is stronger than cancellous bone, but it is much heavier as well. This arrangement of an outer layer of compact bone, supported from the inside by a filling of lighter cancellous bone, gives the optimum balance between strength and weight.

What is bone actually made of?

Like all of the tissues in the body, bone is made of a mixture of cells and extracellular matrix. The bone cells themselves are responsible for producing and maintaining the strong extracellular matrix, which gives bone its structure. The main component of this extracellular matrix, as in most tissues, is **collagen** which is the most abundant protein in the body and has a structure that allows it to be formed into long thin fibres. These fibres are packed together in a very organised manner, which makes the resulting matrix structure very strong (Figure 3.8).

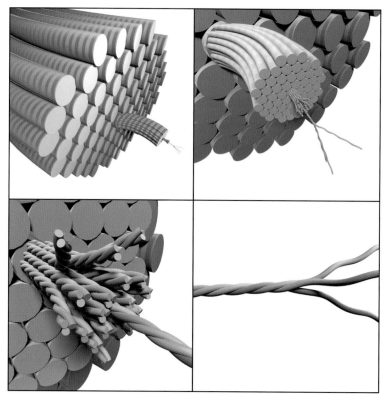

Figure 3.8 Collagen fibres are made from triple helices (three strands twisted together; see bottom right diagram) of protein molecules and can be packed together in a highly organised manner. This schematic diagram shows the organisation of bundles of collagen fibres at increasing magnification; the sequence is viewed along the top row (left to right) and then the bottom row (left to right). (Source: Copyright 2004 Symmation LLC)

A mineral is a crystalline chemical compound which does not contain organic compounds (compounds with carbon-to-carbon (C—C) bonds).

Whilst the *strength* in bone comes from the collagen, the *hardness* is conferred by the mineral component of bone – calcium-containing crystals that are incorporated into the collagen framework. In some ways, bone matrix structure can be compared to reinforced concrete: the collagen fibres are like the metal rods which provide strength and support to the concrete which is poured in and sets to provide the hardness (Figure 3.9). The combination of two materials (collagen and minerals) enables bone to be strong, hard, and resilient. If bones were made from collagen alone, then they would be too flexible; if they were made from minerals only, they would be too brittle.

Of course, unlike reinforced concrete, bone is a living tissue which must grow and be maintained. There are two main cell types involved in maintaining the structure of bone: osteoblasts and osteoclasts (notice they are both called 'osteo' which indicates that they are specifically found in bone). **Osteoblasts** are the bone-forming cells which secrete collagen and organise the mineralisation of bone. **Osteoclasts** disassemble or *resorb* bone in order to remodel it into an optimal shape. A fine balance between the activity of these two cell types maintains normal bone structure and function and allows it to respond to changes during growth or repair.

This balance between bone formation and resorption changes gradually through life. During childhood and early adulthood, there is more formation than resorption. From middle age onwards, the balance shifts gradually so that there is more resorption than formation. Some people suffer from bone diseases in which the balance shifts too far towards resorption of bone and an excessive loss of bone structure results. Such a condition is called **osteoporosis** (literally means having *porous bones*) and leaves sufferers more susceptible to fractures (Figure 3.10).

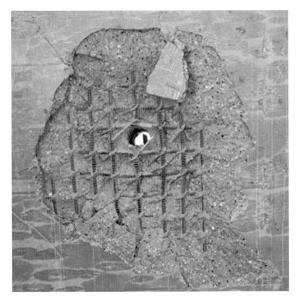

Figure 3.9   Reinforced concrete. (Source: United States Air Force)

Circumstances that may lead to this include periods when bone is subject to reduced loading (as a result of prolonged bed rest, immobilisation or, perhaps less common, when astronauts spend a long time without gravity), changes in hormone levels (in particular reductions in the hormone oestrogen following the menopause in women) and the presence of excess corticosteroid drugs, which can be given as treatments for conditions such as asthma and chronic obstructive pulmonary disease (COPD). Smoking has also been identified as a risk factor for developing osteoporosis (Pathy et al., 2006).

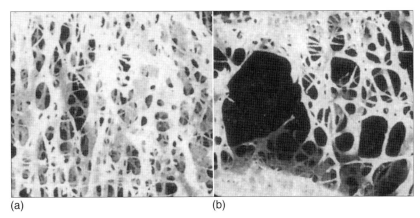

(a)   (b)

Figure 3.10   The structure of (a) normal and (b) osteoporotic bone showing the reduced number of trabeculae, resulting in weaker bones. (Source: International Osteoporosis Foundation)

White cells (leukocytes) circulate through the blood and tissues and are an important component of the immune system which fights infection and disease.

Apart from the hard bone tissue itself, there are two other important structures. In the central region of some larger bones there is **bone marrow**, which contains the specialised cells that make white cells and red blood cells and a variety of other cells. You may have heard of people receiving *bone marrow transplants* following diseases or treatments that reduce the ability of their own bone marrow to produce white cells. Because bone marrow contains *stem cells*, which can continuously divide to form different types of blood cells (and more stem cells), just a few stem cells from a donor can be sufficient to produce all of the cells required in the recipient. Stem cells will be discussed in more detail in Chapter 5.

Bone marrow also contains many fat-storing cells, which supply the components required for stem cell division. It is the fat that gives bone marrow its jelly-like texture, and makes it such a treat for carnivores to eat!

The other structure of interest is the layer of **cartilage** (indicated in Figure 3.4) that coats the ends of the long bones. This is known as *articular* cartilage because it is found at the joints (articulation is another word for joint). It is a specialised tissue which is very smooth and resilient and does not have the mineral components found in bone tissue.

◆ The *structure* of articular cartilage is that of a smooth resilient coating on the ends of the long bones. What *function* do you think this performs?

◆ Articular cartilage provides a smooth surface that reduces friction and protects the bones during joint movement.

A calcium ion is a calcium atom that has lost two negatively charged electrons and therefore possesses two positive charges. It is written Ca^{2+}.

One other important extra role of the bones stems from the fact that they contain so many calcium ions. Crystals containing **calcium ions** are an important mineral element of the bones themselves, but calcium ions are also a vital component of many chemical reactions throughout the body so their concentration in the blood needs to be carefully maintained. The bones can be considered to act as a reservoir for calcium ions: if the calcium levels in the blood drop (perhaps because of insufficient calcium in the diet, or a problem in absorbing it from the gut into the bloodstream) then calcium ions are released from the bones in order to make up the shortfall. The result of this is that bone structure becomes weaker in order to maintain the correct level of calcium ions in the blood.

3.3.2 Muscle

The type of muscle tissue that moves the limbs and will be discussed here is called **skeletal muscle** (muscle that is part of the musculoskeletal system). This distinguishes it from other types of muscle in the body such as cardiac muscle (heart muscle tissue) and smooth muscle (found in structures such as the walls of arteries and the gut). All types of muscle perform the same main function: contraction of the muscle changes its shape and moves the structures to which it is attached. At a fundamental level, muscle tissue converts *chemical* energy (stored in the chemical bonds of molecules) into *kinetic* energy (energy in the form of movement).

In addition to this main function, muscles also convert some chemical energy into heat energy – this is why shivering (repetitive contraction of skeletal muscles) is a useful response to the body being cold.

Muscle tissue, like all tissues, is made up of cells and extracellular matrix. In this case, the cells are highly specialised to suit their contractile function, and their appearance is rather different from other cells you may have studied. The contractile cells are called **myofibres** (or muscle fibres) and are long and thin (as is suggested by the term fibre) and each cell is multinucleated, i.e. it contains more than one nucleus (Figure 3.11).

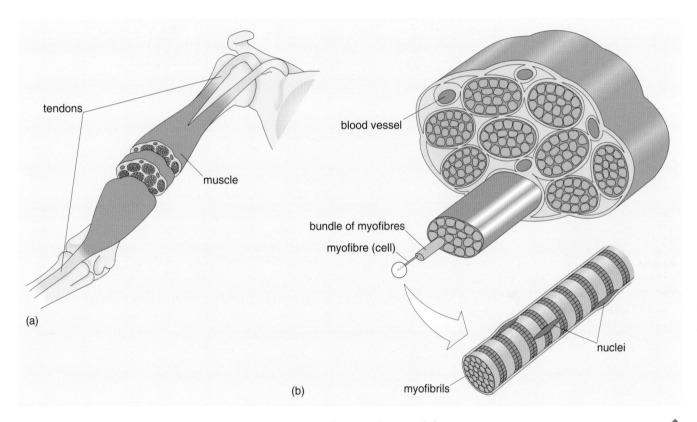

Figure 3.11 (a) Schematic diagram of the structure of a muscle containing many individual myofibres which are (b) single multinucleated cells.

Inside the myofibres are long organelles (Box 3.2 overleaf) called **myofibrils**, which run the full length of the cell and contain the proteins that allow contraction.

This multinucleated structure is unusual (cells normally each contain one nucleus) and is due to the fact that myofibres are formed by joining together lots of other cells (called myoblasts) which then fuse to form one long single cell retaining all the nuclei.

Box 3.2 (Explanation) Organelles

Inside cells there are a large number of individual structures collectively called *organelles* (Figure 3.12). The *nucleus* is the largest organelle and contains the cell's inherited genetic material in the form of DNA. The *mitochondria* (migh-toe-kon-dree-ah) are the organelles that produce the energy that fuels all of the processes that go on in the cell, and the *endoplasmic reticulum* is where new proteins are made.

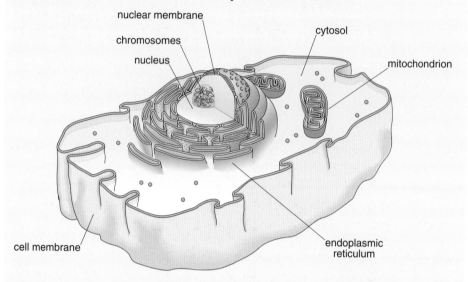

Figure 3.12 A schematic drawing of a cell cut in half to show some of the features that are found in most human cells. Human cells are 10–100 μm across, depending on their type.

◆ Since muscle contraction requires a great deal of energy to be provided from chemical sources such as glucose, what organelles might you expect to find close to the contractile myofibrils?

◆ Mitochondria, the 'powerhouses' of the cell, are where energy is converted into a form that can be used in muscle contraction. Many mitochondria are located throughout myofibres.

Myofibres are packed together in a highly aligned manner within a supporting extracellular matrix and layers of connective tissue to maintain the most efficient arrangement of myofibrils for contraction (Figure 3.13).

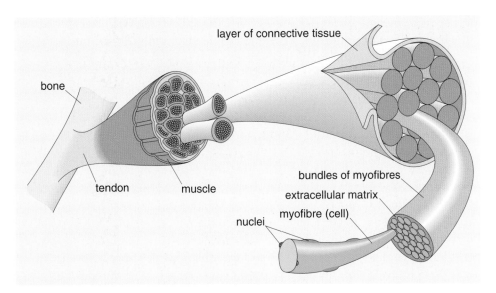

Figure 3.13   Schematic diagram to illustrate the supporting extracellular matrix and layers of connective tissue in skeletal muscles that are continuous with the tendon that connects the muscle to the bone.

The network of collagen that runs throughout the muscle and surrounds the myofibres is gathered together at the ends of the muscle and enables the movement generated by muscle contraction to be transmitted to the bone. The structure that forms from the fibres of the extracellular matrix at the ends of the muscle, and joins the muscle to the bone, is classed as a tissue in its own right – *tendon*.

3.3.3   Tendon

Tendons are like ropes that attach muscles to bones (or sometimes to other muscles). They have a high *tensile strength* (they can withstand being pulled on with great force without breaking) and often have to be flexible enough to bend around joints. They are made from the same extracellular matrix material as the muscles from which they extend (mainly collagen fibres) but are unable to contract like muscles. They are also very resistant to stretching.

The collagen fibres in tendons are highly organised, somewhat like the bundles of fibres within a rope or a steel cable. At the microscopic level, tendons appear to be composed almost entirely of tightly packed and carefully aligned collagen fibres. They also have a small number of elastic fibres present amongst the collagen fibres. You may wonder why a tissue that is resistant to stretching has elastic fibres. When a tendon is put under a very high load, approaching the maximum it can withstand, it stretches very slightly. This protects it from damage, and the recoil (due to the elastic fibres) that follows the slight stretching helps with normal movement.

The overall structure of each tendon depends on its precise function within the body: some are long and thin and travel around joints, whilst others are short and thick or even flattened into a ribbon shape.

◆ Apart from the high tensile strength and flexibility of tendons, what other structural features must be present to enable them to fulfil their function (to enable the muscles to move the bones)?

◆ They must be firmly anchored to both the muscle and the bone, and they must be free to move over the surrounding tissue.

In common with other tissues, tendons have particular *intrinsic* structures which are readily associated with their functions (such as tightly packed collagen fibres to give high tensile strength), but there are other features that are just as essential which are involved in the relationship *between* one tissue and the others around it. For example, it would be useless to have a tendon with a tensile strength that would withstand all of the force a muscle could apply, if the attachment point to the bone at the other end was too weak to withstand such a force. Conversely, if a tendon was not able to slide freely over the other neighbouring tissues (such as the underlying bones, the overlying skin, muscles and other tendons), then its function would be impaired.

Tendons are attached very securely to the muscles and the bones they connect. At the muscle end, this is achieved because the collagen fibres of the tendon are a continuation of those *inside* the muscle (Figure 3.14). At the bone end, the collagen fibres spread out again and are attached securely into the bone in a manner that spreads the load. A number of structures exist in order to enable tendons to move freely over their surroundings. In some places, tendons move inside sheaths, rather like the brake cables on a bicycle, whilst in other places they run over 'pulleys' in order to travel around joints.

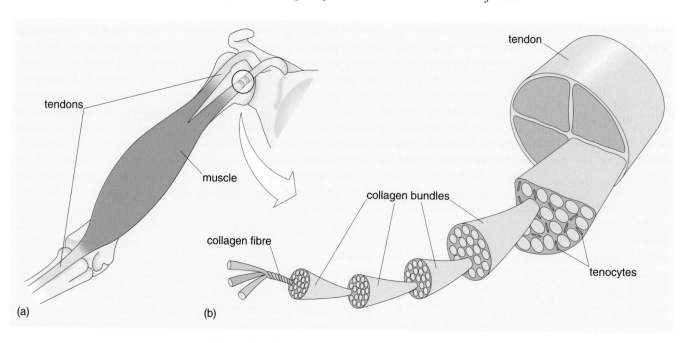

Figure 3.14 Schematic diagrams illustrating (a) tendons showing attachments to muscle and bone and (b) the hierarchical arrangement of fibres in the structure of tendons.

◆ If you clench and unclench your fist as you did in Activity 2.1, you may notice that the finger movement is caused by contraction of muscles in your forearm. Can you describe the path the tendons must take to the bones during this movement?

◆ The tendons must travel down the forearm, through the wrist and hand, then along the fingers.

This is a good example of where tendons need to run through various tunnels and around pulleys to achieve their function (Figure 3.15).

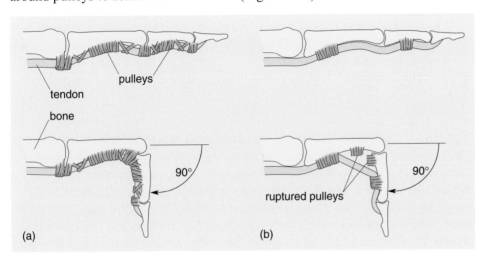

Figure 3.15 Diagram to show (a) how tendons run through pulleys in the hand and (b) what happens when pulleys rupture. (Source: Strickland, 2000, Figure 3)

Whilst tendon structure is dominated by the extracellular matrix, there are cells present whose function is to maintain this living tissue in its healthy form. The cells involved are called *tenocytes* (teen-oh-sites), but adult tendons are sparsely populated with these cells. There are also some blood vessels, but far fewer than in most other tissues.

It is worth mentioning ligaments at this stage, but only briefly. For most purposes, **ligaments** can be considered to be similar in structure to tendons, but instead of connecting muscle to bone they connect bones to each other. This function requires them to be strong, to be well anchored to the bones, and not to stretch very much.

3.3.4 Nerves

All of the nervous system that is not located in the brain and spinal cord forms the *peripheral nervous system* (the brain and spinal cord are the *central nervous system, CNS*). The peripheral nervous system contains specialised cells (neurons) that convey information between the CNS and the rest of the body. The neurons are classified as 'sensory' if they carry information from the body to the CNS and 'motor' if they carry information from the CNS to the muscles. **Neurons** are cells with long structures called axons that project long distances from the cell body, and they communicate with each other through connections called synapses.

When a neuron is stimulated (perhaps by a chemical signal from an adjacent neuron at a synapse, or by a sensation such as pressure or temperature in the skin), an electrical signal travels along the axon (these signals are known as action potentials).

Many neurons, together with other types of cells and extracellular matrix structures, are all bundled together to make a peripheral nerve. An idea of scale is useful here: a neuron is a single cell whose cell body (the round part of the cell that contains the nucleus) is approximately 10 µm across. Its long thin axons are less than 1 µm thick but can be very long since they must connect the cell body of the neuron, which is located close to or within the spinal cord, to parts of the body that could be some distance away.

◈ Can you suggest where in the human body you would find the longest axons? Can you estimate their length?

◆ The longest axons are those that connect the spinal cord to the toes (these are often over a metre long).

Neurons are remarkable cells when you consider that axons can be more than a metre in length but less than a micrometre thick (spare a thought too for the axons in a giraffe that can be many metres long, or in a blue whale tens of metres!). The longest peripheral nerve in the human body is called the sciatic nerve (pronounced 'sigh-attic') which runs down the back of the leg. Clearly some sophisticated support structures are necessary to protect and maintain the delicate axons, particularly when they need to run the length of the limbs, bend and stretch around joints and still conduct action potentials.

The general structure of a peripheral nerve is shown in Figure 3.16.

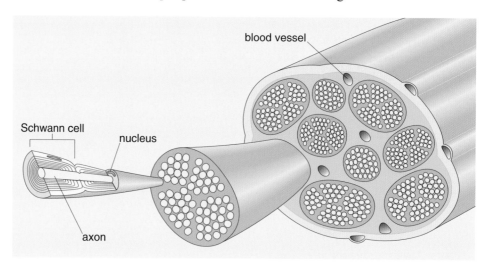

Figure 3.16   A section of peripheral nerve showing axons and Schwann cells.

All the way along its length, each axon is associated with support cells called **Schwann cells** (shwonn). In many cases, the Schwann cells wrap themselves around the axon; this enables faster more efficient transmission of action potentials along the axon. Axons and their Schwann cells are bundled together along with some collagen fibres to provide strength, and are wrapped up in an outer layer containing a protective meshwork of collagen fibres. It is this

10 µm means 10 micrometres; there are 1000 µm in a millimetre.

complete assembly that is referred to as the *nerve* (not to be confused with the individual neurons inside a nerve), and nerves can be many millimetres in diameter (some can be seen by the naked eye and in appearance they are like a white shiny thread). Blood vessels also run throughout the nerves. Some nerves contain bundles of both motor and sensory axons, while some carry just one type.

If the course of a nerve is followed from the spinal cord down a limb, various branch points occur where different axons are directed off to various parts of the body. This gives rise to a peripheral nerve network which runs throughout the body and includes nerve structures with a wide range of dimensions from the thick sciatic nerve at the top of the leg to the thin branches containing a few axons near the toes (Figure 3.17). This branching network resembles a tree and this analogy is useful to bear in mind when considering nerves in the context of traumatic injury. Damage to a thin branch or a twig would not cause much damage to the entire tree, but cutting through the trunk or a major branch would damage everything branching out beyond that point. So in terms of nerve injury, damage to one of the fine branches of the nerves that, for example, give sensation to a small patch of skin on the foot would be easily tolerated, whereas damage to one of the thick nerves near the spinal cord could cause major loss of sensation and muscle function in an entire limb.

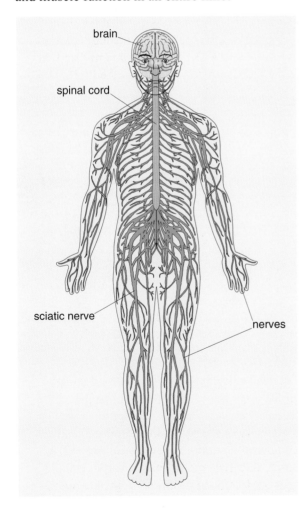

Figure 3.17   The network of peripheral nerves (notice that the nerves get thinner the further away they are from the spinal cord, because they branch off to different areas).

3.3.5 Skin

The principal function of the skin is to act as a barrier to the outside world. It is also a sensory organ (a very large one – the typical skin surface area of an adult is 1.5–2.0 m^2), and it plays an important role in maintaining body temperature. The structure of skin will be described briefly and related to these functions. Later on in this book, the role of skin in healing following traumatic injury will also be discussed, so some understanding of skin structure is important.

Skin contains two main layers: the epidermis, which is the outermost layer, and the underlying dermis (Figure 3.18). Beneath the dermis there is a layer of *subcutaneous* fat (cutaneous, pronounced 'cue-tay-nee-us', refers to the skin; subcutaneous therefore means under the skin).

1 m^2 = 1 square metre, i.e. an area 1 m × 1 m.

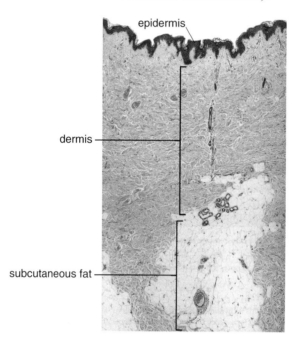

Figure 3.18 The layered structure of skin showing epidermis, dermis and subcutaneous fat. (Source: Lowe et al., 2006)

The **epidermis** forms the outer waterproof protective layer of the skin and varies in thickness according to where it is in the body.

◇ Since the epidermis is a protective layer, where would you expect it to be thickest?

◆ The epidermis is thickest on the palms of the hands and soles of the feet – the areas that require the most protection from constant wear and tear.

The epidermis is quite unlike the other tissues that have been discussed so far, since it is predominantly made from dead cells and contains no blood vessels or nerve endings. The base layer of the epidermis does contain some live cells, which are able to divide and produce new cells to form the epidermis. Once produced, these cells (called keratinocytes (kare-atin-oh-sites)) are gradually pushed towards the surface of the epidermis as more new cells are formed beneath them. As they move outwards, they become flat and a fibrous protein called keratin is made inside the cells (hence the cell name). As the keratinocytes reach the outer layers of the epidermis they die, so these outer layers are made from lots of flat thin dead cells packed full of keratin. These outer dead cells are constantly being rubbed off and are replaced by the continuous stream of newly formed cells moving outwards. It takes about 40 days for complete replacement

A large part of household dust is actually dead keratinocytes!

of the epidermis through this process. As well as containing the cells that divide to give rise to the keratinocytes, the base layer of the epidermis contains other cell types including those that give the skin its colour (pigment) and provide chemicals to protect the skin from the harmful effects of the sun.

The **dermis** lies immediately beneath the epidermis and is far more reminiscent of the other tissues described so far.

◆ What are the general features of tissues?

◆ They tend to have living cells embedded within an extracellular matrix containing proteins such as collagen, with blood capillaries to supply oxygen and nutrients.

The dermis provides the strength of skin, making it sufficiently robust and elastic to fulfil its protective function. These physical properties come from the extracellular matrix proteins, which are strong collagen fibres interlaced with elastic protein fibres. There are a number of different cell types present in the dermis. *Fibroblasts* produce and maintain the extracellular matrix proteins, and there are also immune system cells present throughout the skin, ready to respond to damage, invading microbes or other harmful substances. Throughout the dermis, there are capillaries and sensory nerve endings. Underlying the dermis, there are fat cells which store energy in the form of fat but also serve to cushion and insulate the body. The dermis also contains sweat glands and hairs, both of which are involved in the temperature regulation function of the skin (Figure 3.19).

Figure 3.19 The layered structure of skin showing (a) epithelial cells in the epidermis; (b) connective tissue; (c) muscle; (d) epithelial cells lining a sweat duct; (e) subcutaneous fat.

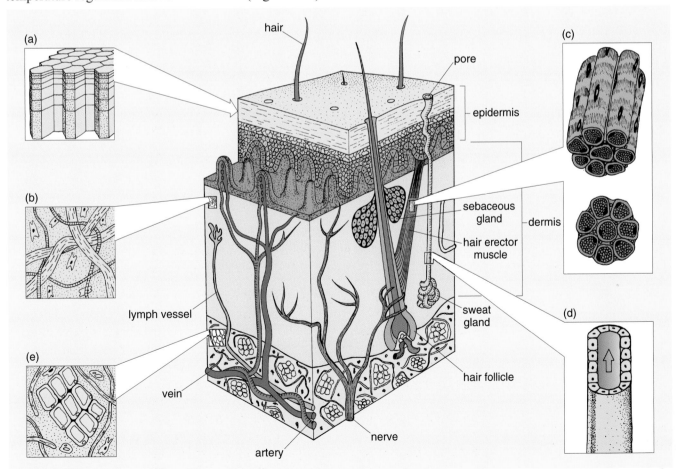

Sweat glands are ducts lined with *epithelial cells* which originate in the subcutaneous tissue and open onto the surface of the skin or into the hair follicles. Sweat is a salty fluid that is released by the sweat glands in response to nerve signals (triggered by fear or excessive heat) – the sweat evaporates from the surface of the skin using heat energy, thus helping to cool the body down. Hairs are formed in the hair follicles which contain keratinocytes that, just like in the epidermis, are pushed outwards and undergo a cycle of keratin production and cell death to produce a hair. Hairs have tiny muscles attached to their base, which can contract in response to nerve signals and make the hair stand up straight (when these muscles are relaxed, the hair lies flat on the surface of the skin). This muscle contraction also makes the skin around the hair muscle bulge, giving rise to 'goose pimples'.

◆ Making the hairs on the skin stand up straight traps a layer of air next to the skin. What function might this serve?

◆ Air is a good insulator, and a layer of air helps to prevent heat loss from the body (in much the same way as a layer of clothing traps warm air next to the skin).

3.3.6 Blood vessels

As described in Chapter 2, the cardiovascular system moves oxygenated blood around the body through the arteries by contraction of the heart, then brings the deoxygenated blood back to the heart via the veins. Within the tissues, the arteries branch into a network of narrow capillaries. In the capillaries, the blood is under less pressure than in the arteries and moves more slowly. The walls of the capillaries are very thin, which allows some of the fluid to leak out of the blood into the surrounding tissues, where it is then known as *tissue fluid* or extracellular fluid. The red blood cells and large dissolved blood plasma proteins remain inside the capillaries, but the tissue fluid allows dissolved nutrients and oxygen to reach the tissue cells via diffusion. All of the cells within a tissue are bathed in the tissue fluid, and the network of capillaries ensures that all cells are close to a supply of oxygen and nutrients.

◆ The leakage of water into the tissues will leave the blood in the capillaries with a reduced water content. Can you suggest how this imbalance might be redressed?

◆ Tissue fluid moves back into the capillaries, redressing the balance. This means that there is a continuous exchange of fluid between the inside of the capillaries and the surrounding tissue cells (Figure 3.20).

About 90% of the tissue fluid actually re-enters capillaries; the other 10% drains into the lymphatic system which is a network of ducts that collects the tissue fluid and eventually directs it back into the blood circulation.

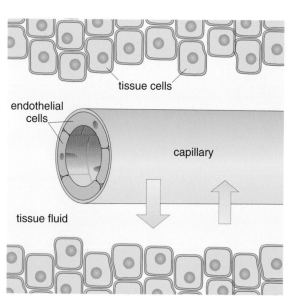

tissue cells

endothelial cells

capillary

tissue fluid

Figure 3.20 Fluid movement between capillaries and tissue.

The walls of capillaries are composed of **endothelial cells** (end-oh-thee-lee-al); these are flat cells that line the entire cardiovascular system like the tiles on the inside wall of a tunnel.

In capillaries, the walls of the vessels are made of one thin layer of endothelial cells. As you might have predicted, the cells are surrounded by extracellular matrix which holds them in place. In larger vessels the inner lining has additional layers of tissue providing strength and durability, and some have a layer of smooth muscle cells which can contract or relax to alter the internal dimensions of the blood vessel (causing constriction or dilation) (look back at Figure 2.3b). This effect is seen during *vasodilation* (vay-zoh) and *vasoconstriction* of the blood vessels supplying the capillaries in the dermis. During vasodilation, blood flow to the dermis increases and the skin turns red; during vasoconstriction, the blood flow to the dermis decreases and the skin turns pale. This function is used for cooling the body (vasodilation) or conserving body heat by reducing blood flow through the skin (vasoconstriction).

The word *endothelium* (plural: endothelia) is used to refer to this interface between the blood inside the vessels and the tissues of the body. It should not be confused with the word *epithelium* (plural epithelia) which refers to the interface between the body tissues and the outside world (for example, the outer surface of the skin, the lining of the gut and the lining of ducts and glands such as mammary glands are all *epi*thelia).

3.4 Limb architecture and trauma mechanics

So far, this chapter has discussed the various individual components that make up a limb – bones, muscles, tendons, nerves and skin, each with their specific arrangement of cells and extracellular matrix, and all bathed in oxygen and nutrients supplied from blood capillaries. However, studying these tissues in isolation is rather artificial, since in the body they are intricately arranged together to provide a functional system. It is important to consider the *interfaces* between the different tissues in order to understand their relationships. For example, the interfaces between the end of a muscle, a tendon and a bone need to provide a very strong anchoring point in order to ensure that the force generated by the muscle is transferred efficiently to move the bone. On the other hand, along the length of the same muscle where it runs parallel to the bone, the surfaces of the different tissues must have no attachment at all, otherwise when the muscle moved, tearing and tissue damage would result (Figure 3.21).

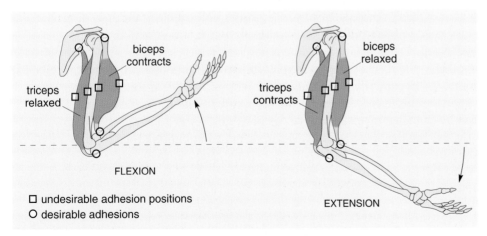

Figure 3.21 Muscle contraction showing movement of limb and of muscles to illustrate the location of desirable and undesirable adhesions.

This organisation of tissues to enable them to be securely anchored together in some places, yet able to move freely over each other in other locations, is fundamental to understanding normal function and is also very important in understanding damage and repair (Activity 3.1).

Activity 3.1 The arrangement of tissues in the leg

Allow about 1 hour

Activity 3.1 is a multimedia exercise on the DVD associated with this book which will enable you to delve into the three-dimensional architecture of the leg. You will be able to look in detail at representations of the individual tissues, stripping them away layer by layer, but you should also spend some time getting a feel for how the various components interact with each other in a three-dimensional manner in order to fulfil their functions.

If you are unable to complete this activity now, do so as soon as possible; you may find it more difficult to study the rest of this chapter until you have done so.

Sometimes it is useful to step back from the biology of tissue structure and function and consider the human body in the way that an engineer might consider a structure such as a bridge or a building – a complex arrangement of different materials interacting to perform a function.

Medical staff sometimes apply this kind of approach following traumatic injuries, by thinking about how the forces that have been exerted on the body might cause damage. An example would be a person who has fallen from a height – if he or she landed on their feet, then the force of the impact could be transmitted up the body through the long bones (rigid material that transfers force), so staff would suspect the possibility of compression fractures occurring perhaps in the spine, some distance from the site of impact (the feet). However, if the person had landed flat then distant compression fractures of this kind would be less likely to occur than more localised damage to the parts of the body near the impact. Bones transfer forces because they are rigid materials (they need to be in order to fulfil their support function within the body), but this also means that they do not deform much when excessive forces are applied to them. They deform slightly up to a certain threshold amount of force, but beyond this limit they break (see Box 3.3). Softer tissues such as skin and muscle can deform to a greater extent without breaking, but they can be damaged by excessive forces nonetheless (soft tissues can be torn or crushed and the blood vessels within them can be ruptured, disrupting the blood supply).

Box 3.3 (Enrichment) Bones as materials

Bones are capable of deforming slightly under load and then returning to their original shape in an *elastic* manner. This enables them to sustain forces that deform them by up to about 0.5% of their original length (this is known as a 0.5% strain). However, if they are subjected to forces that deform them by more than about 0.5%, then they can be permanently damaged, and at deformation approaching 3% they break. Figure 3.22 shows the stress–strain curve for a typical long bone where stress is the amount of force per unit area applied to the bone and strain is its relative change in size (deformation). As stress increases along the vertical axis, the strain along the horizontal axis increases in a linear manner (straight line) until approximately 0.5%. So, up to this point, the increase in stress is matched by a proportionate increase in strain. Increases beyond this point result in much larger deformations which are permanent and, if they reach 3%, the bone breaks.

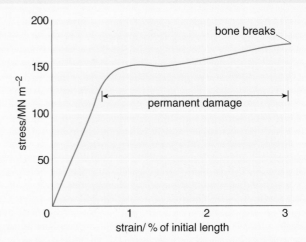

Figure 3.22 A line graph showing the stress–strain curve for a typical long bone. The units of stress and strain are given in MN m^{-2} (mega newtons per square metre).

People who have been involved in traffic accidents are frequently exposed to large forces because of the speeds involved before impact. Impact transfers the *kinetic* energy (movement energy) of a moving vehicle into other forms of energy, mainly forces causing deformation of structures such as the parts of the vehicle (Figure 3.23). If a moving car strikes a pedestrian, then some of this kinetic energy is transferred to forces that deform the previously stationary tissues of the person who has been hit. However, a passenger in a car that crashes as in Figure 3.23 experiences more complex forces. As the moving vehicle stops, the passenger will keep moving forward until they are restrained by a seat belt or until they hit part of the car interior (airbags are designed to cushion passengers at this stage). This rapid deceleration will cause direct impact injuries such as those experienced by the pedestrian; but this time, rapidly moving parts of the body come into contact with stationary parts of the car. Finally, during rapid deceleration, the internal organs (e.g. the stomach and the brain) collide with the internal structures of the body (e.g. the ribs and the skull). Like the passenger, such organs will continue moving forward until restrained by internal structures, at which point there will be an internal impact and organ damage.

Figure 3.23 Set of still images showing a crash test in which a car impacts a solid wall, revealing what happens to the structure of the vehicle and the 'dummy' passengers. Photographs (a) to (c) have been taken in sequence at intervals of a fraction of a second. Simulations such as this enable the forces that affect the human body in the event of a collision to be predicted. (Source: TRL Ltd/Science Photo Library)

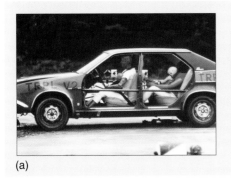

(a)

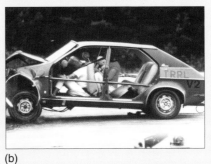

(b)

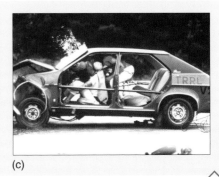

(c)

By thinking about the mechanics of an accident, medical staff are able to direct their investigations towards the most likely types of injury. For example, someone who was in a car crash involving rapid deceleration or acceleration (for example, hitting, or being hit by, another car) is most likely to have sustained a neck injury, due to the 'whiplash' effect of the unrestrained head moving rapidly back and forth while the body is held in place by the seat and seat belt. Understanding the body as a mechanical structure is a complex area known as *biomechanics* which enables predictions to be made about how tissues may be damaged in the event of trauma. The following quotation comes from one of the paramedics (Figure 3.24) you saw in DVD Activity 2.2a and is included to illustrate how paramedics would think about the mechanics of an accident:

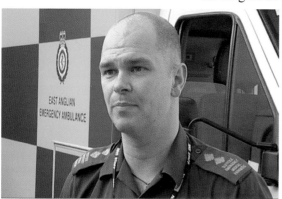

Figure 3.24 A paramedic with the East Anglian Ambulance Service, who was part of the team demonstrating the removal of an injured passenger from a car in DVD Activity 2.2a. (Source: Owen Horn/Open University)

'There are calculations that are required to be undertaken at the scene of an accident…working out what kinetic energy has been transferred…how fast the vehicle may have been travelling. The faster the speed, the more kinetic energy has been transferred…and that's half the mass times velocity squared.'

Summary of Chapter 3

3.1 The musculoskeletal system involves a number of separate tissues working together in order to provide coordinated functions. The tissues are arranged to allow movement, with muscles working as antagonistic pairs and bones working as levers.

3.2 A lever rotating around a fulcrum enables a force to be amplified (e.g. a worker lifting a rock) or a distance to be amplified (e.g. in the arm when a small movement of the biceps muscle results in a large movement of the forearm).

3.3 All tissues are composed of cells and extracellular matrix.

3.4 Long bones are made from compact and cancellous bone; compact bone is denser and stronger than cancellous bone and the two are arranged in a way that provides a compromise between strength and weight. Bone extracellular matrix is composed of strong collagen fibres and hard calcium-containing crystals. It is continuously maintained and remodelled by the action of osteoblasts and osteoclasts.

3.5 Skeletal muscles contract to enable movement. Myofibres are long thin multinucleated cells containing contractile myofibrils and many mitochondria which generate the energy for movement.

3.6 The collagen fibres that run through muscles continue out of the ends of the muscle and form the tendons that attach muscles to bones. Tendons have a high tensile strength and are resistant to stretching. They contain only a few cells and some blood vessels but are predominantly made from extracellular matrix (especially collagen).

3.7 Peripheral nerves are a branching network of bundles of axons (the long thin extensions of single neurons) which connect all parts of the body to the central nervous system. The axons are associated with Schwann cells and the bundles of axons with their Schwann cells are arranged within an outer layer formed from extracellular matrix.

3.8 Skin is a protective barrier, a sensory organ, and it plays a role in temperature control. The outer layers of the epidermis are dead keratinocytes, which are constantly replenished by cell division in the innermost layers. Beneath the epidermis is the dermis which contains many cells, extracellular matrix and blood vessels. Sweat glands, hair follicles and subcutaneous fat are also important skin components.

3.9 Blood vessels branch to form capillaries which supply the cells within tissues with oxygen and nutrients. Blood flow can be controlled by contraction of the smooth muscle in the walls of blood vessels. Tissue fluid leaks out of the capillaries, which have thin walls lined with endothelial cells. The fluid bathes the tissue cells before returning to the capillaries or collecting in the lymphatic system for returning to the blood circulation.

3.10 Tissues are intimately arranged within body structures such as the limbs, acting together to provide coordinated function. Some interfaces between tissues are very strong (e.g. tendon attachment to bone) and others provide free movement (where tissues must move past each other).

Learning outcomes for Chapter 3

After studying this chapter and its associated activities, you should be able to:

LO 3.1 Define and use in context, or recognise definitions and applications of, each of the terms printed in **bold** in the text. (Question 3.1 and 3.4)

LO 3.2 Demonstrate an understanding that the combined interaction of various different tissues enables musculoskeletal system function. (Questions 3.3 and 3.4 and DVD Activity 3.1)

LO 3.3 Describe how forces (from muscles) are conducted through tendons and bones to result in a simple limb movement. (Question 3.4 and DVD Activity 3.1)

LO 3.4 Describe how the musculoskeletal system uses the principles of levers in limb movement, and calculate the forces and distances in lever systems. (Questions 3.4 and 3.5 and Activity C1 for Open University students)

LO 3.5 Describe the key features of the six tissues (bone, muscle, nerve, tendon, skin, blood vessels) typically damaged during a traumatic limb injury and relate their structure to function. (Questions 3.1, 3.2 and 3.4 and DVD Activity 3.1)

LO 3.6 Discuss the importance of different types of interfaces between tissues that enable a limb to function (anchoring points and gliding surfaces). (Questions 3.3 and 3.4)

Self-assessment questions for Chapter 3

Question 3.1 (LOs 3.1 and 3.5)

Briefly describe which structures in skin are related to the functions of (a) protection, (b) sensation and (c) temperature regulation.

Question 3.2 (LO 3.5)

Since tendons are made predominantly of similar extracellular matrix fibres (collagen) to those found in muscles and bones, why are they not stiff like bones or contractile like muscles?

Question 3.3 (LOs 3.2 and 3.6)

Give two examples of places in the leg where tissues must
(a) adhere strongly to one another and (b) glide past each other.

Question 3.4 (LOs 3.1 to 3.6)

Describe the sequence of musculoskeletal events involved in kicking a ball. Start with a nerve impulse to a muscle and finish with the sensory nerve impulse that detects foot contact with the ball. At each stage, describe the structure and function of the tissue involved.

Question 3.5 (LO 3.4)

Figure 3.25 shows a diagram of a person holding 3 kg exercise weights (the fulcrum is 60 cm from the weight). The downwards force of one of the 3 kg objects is 30 newtons (N). Calculate the force (in N) that will be generated at point X in the tissues (2 cm to the left of the fulcrum). Assume the arm with elbow straight is a simple lever that extends to point X.

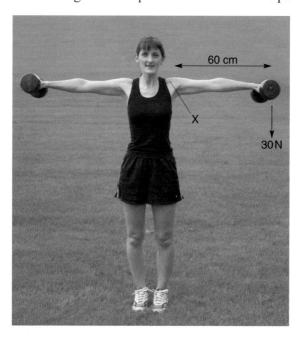

Figure 3.25 A person holding 3 kg weights. (Source: James Phillips)

CHAPTER 4

FRACTURES

In this chapter, some typical 'clinical interventions' will be discussed. These are the procedures that might be carried out in order to prevent an injury from getting worse, and to improve the chances of good repair and rapid recovery. This will be followed by a discussion of fractures caused by falls, particularly in older people who are most prone to falling, with consideration of why they occur and how they might be prevented.

4.1   Severe fractures

Initial medical attention following traumatic injury focuses on any life-threatening damage, as discussed in Chapter 2. Following this initial care, tests are carried out to establish the extent of tissue damage; then an appropriate course of treatment is devised. We turn once more to Hassan who injured his leg in a road traffic accident and was taken to Aga Khan University Hospital in Karachi (Vignette 4.1).

Vignette 4.1   Hassan's leg injury is investigated

Following examination, it was clear to the medical staff that Hassan had probably sustained a broken femur. The femur is the largest bone in the body and is very strong and it would therefore require a substantial force to break it. During the initial stages of assessment, medical staff think about the mechanics of an injury. For example, to produce a fracture of the shaft of the femur in a young fit person would require the kinds of large forces generated in high-speed vehicle accidents or falls from a height.

In order to ascertain the extent of the damage to Hassan's leg, a series of tests were carried out. The pain and swelling in his thigh, as well as some skin lesions (cuts and abrasions), indicated the area of trauma and the staff decided to take X-ray images of the area to investigate the fracture.

In addition to the bone damage that can be detected using X-ray images, damage to other tissues is investigated in a case such as Hassan's. For example, in order to detect whether severe damage to the blood circulation has occurred, staff will check for a pulse further down the leg, and will check skin colour in the feet.

◆ What would these tests show?

◆ A pulse in the knee or ankle would show that arterial blood was flowing through the damaged area, and a normal skin colour would show that venous return was not impaired (see Chapter 2).

If damage to the circulation in this area is suspected, then a surgical procedure would be urgently required to repair the damaged blood vessels. Not only could this damage lead to blood loss and hypovolaemic shock (Section 2.2), but if blood isn't getting through, then the tissues in the lower leg and foot (which may have escaped injury in the initial accident) will die.

◆ How might staff investigate whether the nerves that run through the thigh have been damaged by the accident?

◆ They would check for sensation and control of movement in the lower leg and foot.

Following X-ray examination, hospital staff will be able to decide the best course of action for treating Hassan's injury. Any structural break in bone tissue continuity is referred to as a **fracture**. Fractures are divided into the following types (Figure 4.1):

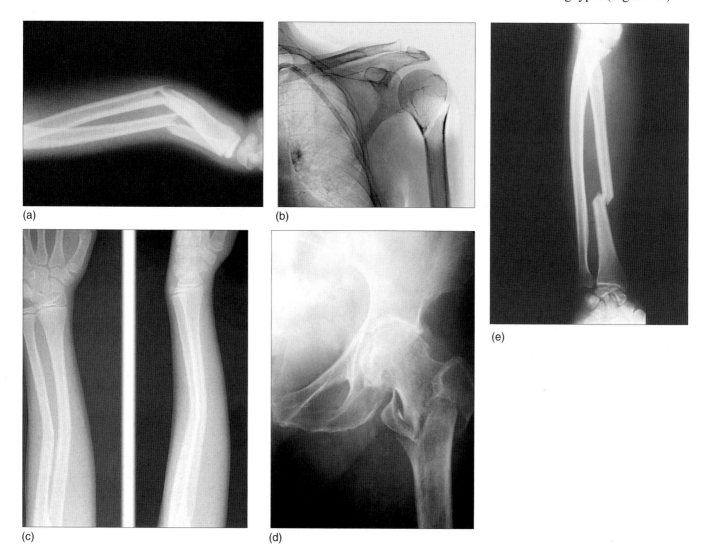

(a)

(b)

(c)

(d)

(e)

Figure 4.1 X-ray images showing some typical types of fracture. (a) An open fracture of the forearm (the hand is to the right); both the fractured long bones have sharp broken ends and part of the broken radius (the upper bone) protrudes through the skin. (Source: Bates, Custom Medical Stock Photo/Science Photo Library). (b) A closed fracture of the upper arm bone (humerus), just below the head of the bone – the broken bone does not penetrate the skin; (note: this image has been enhanced to make the fracture at the top of the bone clearer). (Source: Du Cane Medical Imaging Ltd/Science Photo Library). (c) A greenstick fracture and bowing of both the bones in the forearm (radius and ulna) of a child. (Source: Medical-on-Line/Alamy). (d) An insufficiency fracture in an older woman with osteoporosis where the upper part of the femur has collapsed due to a weakness in bone structure. (Source: Princess Margaret Rose Orthopaedic Hospital/Science Photo Library). (e) An example of a displaced fracture of the radius in the forearm (the hand is at the bottom) where the broken ends of the bone overlap (this is in contrast to an undisplaced fracture of which (b) is an example). (Source: James Stevenson/Science Photo Library)

Open fracture: This is where the overlying skin has been broken and the broken bone is exposed to the outside world.

Closed fracture: The skin remains intact.

Greenstick fracture: An incomplete fracture that often occurs in children whose bones tend to bend rather than break completely (this will be discussed further in Vignette 4.2).

Insufficiency fracture: This is damage caused by 'normal' forces acting on osteoporotic bone.

The severity of a fracture depends on its position and the extent of damage. If the broken parts of the bone are in the correct position (*undisplaced*), then little intervention is required other than immobilising and protecting the damaged area. However, if the fracture is *displaced*, then an operation will often be required in order to realign the broken parts of the bone. A range of fixation devices can be used to hold the broken pieces of bone in the correct position (Figure 4.2).

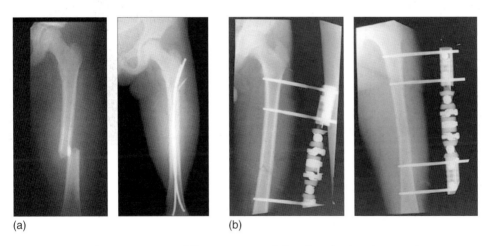

(a)   (b)

Figure 4.2   There are many different types of fixation device that can be tailored to a wide range of fractures. They tend to be made from metal and hold the pieces of fractured bone in the correct position for repair. (a) X-ray images showing realignment of a child's displaced femur fracture using long flexible nails inside the bone. (Source: American Academy of Orthopaedic Surgeons). (b) X-ray images showing realignment of a child's fractured femur using an external fixation device that lies outside the leg and attaches to the bone via long pins. (Source: Flynn, 1998)

As will be discussed in the next chapter, bone has a remarkable capacity for repair. However, the damaged parts of the bone must be held in the correct position in order for the repair to be effective. For a small bone, such as in a finger or toe, it is normally sufficient to **splint** the bone: immobilise it with a piece of rigid material or by taping it to the neighbouring finger or toe. The idea is that the splint provides support – it adopts the mechanical function that the intact bone normally plays, immobilising the damaged area and shielding the repair site from mechanical forces until such time as it has fully repaired. In larger bones, such as those in the arm and the lower part of the leg, a **cast** fulfils a similar function. This hard shell provides protection to the repair site and immobilises the area so that the damaged ends of the fractured bone can fuse.

This rigid support both protects the area from external forces, and also withstands the forces that normally act on bones during normal movement of the muscles.

Vignette 4.2   Hassan is diagnosed as having a broken femur

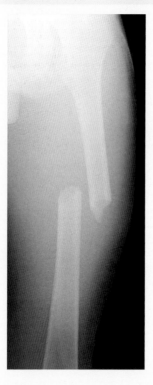

Hassan's X-rays showed that he had indeed sustained a displaced fracture to his femur (Figure 4.3).

Luckily, despite extensive swelling, there were no signs of damage to the circulation or nerves in Hassan's leg. This meant that doctors were able to concentrate on repairing the bone damage. The skin was broken above the fracture site, making this an *open fracture*, so hospital staff were careful to clean the area very thoroughly and administered antibiotics in order to reduce the risk of an infection.

Figure 4.3   Hassan's X-ray showing his fractured femur. Note how the broken ends of the bone overlap. (Source: Phillip Parkinson, Leeds Teaching Hospital NHS Trust)

◆ In Figure 4.3, what forces are acting on the broken femur in Hassan's X-ray to cause the broken ends of the bone to overlap?

◆ The muscles that run alongside the femur will tend to pull the two halves of the broken bone towards each other.

This overlap (Figure 4.3) will interfere with the repair because it stops the broken ends from meshing with each other in their normal position. In such cases, it is often necessary to apply forces to the ends of the broken bone to pull them apart and oppose the tension generated by the muscles. This may be done transiently in order to seat the damaged bones in the appropriate position, or a sustained force (*traction*) might be required to hold them there for a long period (Vignette 4.3).

In many parts of the world, a person sustaining an injury such as Hassan's might have a different experience (Vignette 4.4).

Vignette 4.3 Treatment of Hassan's fracture

Hassan was kept in hospital and wires were put through his femur in order to apply external traction to the site of damage. Figure 4.4 is an X-ray image showing the wire in the lower part of the femur (just above the knee) to which force was applied. Hassan remained in traction in hospital for 6 weeks, after which time his fracture had healed sufficiently to enable the traction to be discontinued and his leg to be put in a cast. This allowed him some mobility (he was able to return home) and protected the repair site for another 6 weeks, after which time the cast was removed. By then, his femur had repaired sufficiently to support his weight during normal movement.

Hassan experienced a very serious fracture caused by a traumatic injury. However, he was fortunate enough to receive expert medical care in a well-equipped hospital, which stabilised his injuries and enabled him to recover.

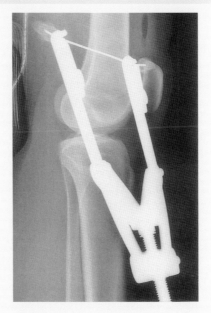

Figure 4.4 An X-ray image showing Hassan's traction fixator. (Source: Radiological Society of North America)

Vignette 4.4 Infection following an open fracture

Shoaib is a similar age to Hassan and lives in a small village in an agricultural area of Pakistan. He experienced a very similar injury to Hassan, an open fracture to his femur. He survived the initial injury and was bandaged up and treated for shock by his family, but it took 2 days before he received medical attention.

◆ What problems do you think this delay could cause to Shoaib?

◆ Because it is an open fracture, without careful cleaning and antibiotic treatment there is a high risk of infection setting in.

By the time Shoaib reached hospital, he was very sick. Not only had he experienced severe pain due to a lack of immobilisation of the injury, made worse by a long bumpy journey, but he was also suffering from a severe infection which damaged the tissues in his leg. By the time he reached the hospital, the damage to the tissues in his leg was so severe that it could not be repaired and the only course was for the leg to be amputated in order to prevent the infection spreading to the rest of his body.

Amputation (removal) of a limb sometimes occurs directly as a result of the traumatic injury, and subsequent surgical amputation is inevitable after very severe injuries which cause so much tissue damage that it would be impossible for any repair to take place. In particular, severe crush injuries which cause damage to large areas of tissue frequently result in amputations. In Vignette 4.4, the amputation was necessary because infection had entered the tissues due to the open fracture breaching the skin, which would normally provide a barrier to prevent the entry of harmful bacteria (Box 4.1). Amputations as a result of infections are more common in places where people have less access to expert medical facilities (as illustrated by the differences in outcome between Hassan and Shoaib whose initial injuries were similar). Where there are problems such as severe damage to the blood circulation in a limb (as checked for during Hassan's hospital examination), then patients without access to surgeons skilled in repairing such damage stand little chance of keeping the limb.

Box 4.1 (Enrichment) Wound infections

Two of the nastiest infections that can result in limb loss and death are *gas gangrene* and *tetanus*.

Gas gangrene is caused by the *Clostridium perfringens* bacterium, which can infect tissues at a site of trauma or surgical wound and release toxins (poisons). The onset can be sudden and dramatic and the damage can spread rapidly. One of the toxins produced by this bacterium is a *collagenase* enzyme which, as the name suggests, breaks down collagen in the tissues with disastrous consequences.

Tetanus is caused by another bacterium called *Clostridium tetani* which releases a toxin that causes paralysis of muscles and can therefore lead to breathing (ventilation) failure and death. In affluent countries, this is now very rare due to an extensive programme of immunisation.

4.2 Greenstick fracture

'Greenstick' fractures are so named because they resemble the fracture that occurs when someone tries to break a fresh green stick from a tree. When an old dry stick is broken, it snaps cleanly into two separate parts, whereas the green stick will bend, then fracture on one side only. Greenstick fractures are often seen in children. This is because their bones have the ability to bend more without breaking than the bones of adults (Vignette 4.5).

◆ Can you suggest what components of the bone determine whether it snaps or bends when force is applied?

◆ The composition of the extracellular matrix, in particular the relative amounts of collagen (strength) and minerals (hardness).

Vignette 4.5   Greenstick fracture (Oliver)

When Oliver was five years old, he was playing in the garden in a toy car, when it toppled over. He put his arm out of the window to break his fall and landed heavily on his hand. He screamed in pain and when his mother dashed out to help him she could see that Oliver's forearm was already looking red and swollen. His mum wrapped some ice cubes in a cloth and held it over the swelling and after a while Oliver stopped crying, but was restless and cried out if his arm was moved. His mother could just about feel an unusual and painful lump in the forearm near his wrist, so she took Oliver to the Accident and Emergency Department of the local hospital.

Oliver was sent to the X-ray department and he and his mother put on lead aprons to protect them from unnecessary radiation. His mother cuddled him while three X-rays were taken of his arm from different angles. Later a doctor showed them the X-ray films (Figure 4.5), and pointed out the bent region known as a greenstick fracture in Oliver's *radius* (the larger of the two bones in the forearm). Oliver's forearm and elbow were put in a cast to keep them immobilised for the next six weeks (Figure 4.6). He went home the same night. For the next two days, he was given analgesic syrup four times a day to help ease the pain, and he gradually got used to wearing the cast. When it was removed he was soon back to normal activity and his arm had completely healed.

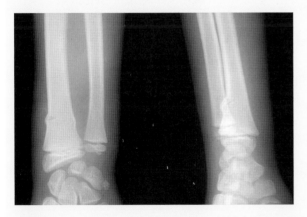

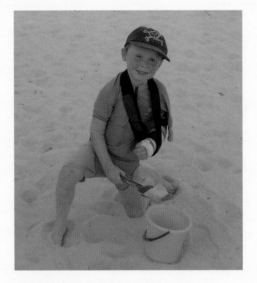

Figure 4.5   X-rays of a forearm (left, front view and right, side view) with a greenstick fractured radius near the wrist. You can see the bulge where the bone has bent under the impact of the fall and is only partly fractured on one side. (Source: Phototake Inc./Photolibrary)

Figure 4.6   Oliver with his arm in a cast. (Source: Johanna Pichowski)

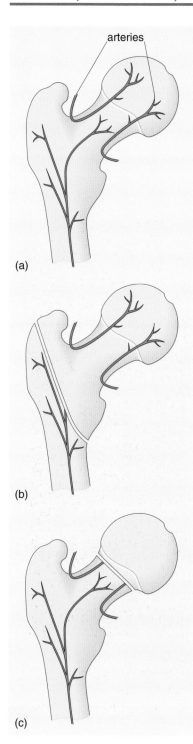

arteries

(a)

(b)

(c)

Figure 4.9 The position of the typical sites of hip fracture, showing (a) the normal blood supply to the head of the femur, (b) that the blood supply is maintained if the fracture is low down but (c) is cut off if the fracture is higher.

4.3 Fractured hip

The hip is a 'ball and socket' joint which is formed where the top of the femur (the ball) meets the pelvis (the socket) (Figure 4.7).

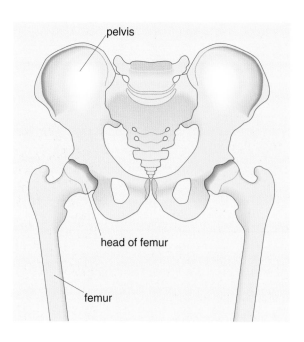

pelvis

head of femur

femur

Figure 4.7 The hip joint is where the head of the femur meets the pelvis. The pelvis bones form cup-shaped sockets into which the ball-shaped heads of the tops of the femurs fit.

Fractures to the hip are relatively common, especially in older people, and usually involve the femur breaking near the ball. There are certain places in this region where fractures typically occur, shown in Figure 4.8.

Whilst the subtly different positions of these fractures may seem a rather obscure thing to focus on, they are actually critical in terms of treatment and, more importantly in the context of this book, are important in understanding the biology of bone repair.

The reason why the position of the fracture is so important concerns the blood supply to this part of the bone, which is shown in Figure 4.9a. If the fracture occurs low down (Figure 4.9b) then the blood supply to the top of the bone (head of femur) is maintained. However, if the fracture occurs higher up (Figure 4.9c) then the blood supply to the head of the femur is impaired and this part of the bone will deteriorate and collapse. In this way, the position of the fracture will determine whether it will be sufficient to align the damaged parts or whether the head of the femur might need to be replaced.

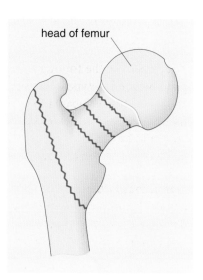

head of femur

Figure 4.8 The typical sites at the top of the femur where fractures to the hip tend to occur.

◆ Why will the head of the femur deteriorate without a good blood supply?

◆ Bone is a living tissue containing cells that maintain it in a healthy state. If these cells are starved of blood, they will die and the surrounding extracellular matrix will not be maintained and so will deteriorate.

Vignette 4.6 describes a skiing accident that resulted in a fracture to the femur.

Vignette 4.6   A skiing accident

It felt like I flew up in the air before I crashed down on the ice. I hit the ground hard but, mercifully, I wasn't tangled up with my skis and nothing hurt. So I thought that I couldn't have broken any bones, though I guessed I'd have spectacular bruising. A few deep breaths, then I accepted the offer of help and was pulled back onto my feet. So far fine, but as I turned I found myself sitting on the ice again. My leg wouldn't support me. By now the 'blood wagon' had been called and within minutes I was being strapped into a stretcher and expertly transported to a wooden hut to await an ambulance. Within an hour of the accident I was in a small basement room in a nearby hospital about to have a 'drip' stuck into me. 'What's that for?' I demanded. 'It's a painkiller', I was told. 'But I have no pain', I replied. 'Good, we'll keep it that way'. And they did. As I was wheeled away after an X-ray that had revealed a bad break to the neck of the femur (Figure 4.10), I noticed posters on the corridor walls: '*This is a pain-free environment*' – and it was!

They operated the following day, fitting a compression plate, which is a type of internal fixation device. It took two and a half hours apparently: still no pain although the soft tissues were very bruised and the knee was 'frozen', quite unable to move. The physiotherapist was along the next day and gave me some exercises.

Unfortunately the leg is now 10 mm shorter than previously and the bone took 10 months to heal. Two years later, despite regular exercise, the muscles in the left leg are weak and I walk with a limp. But no pain!

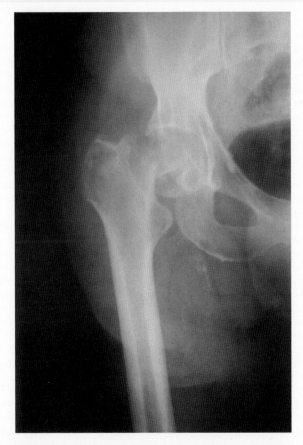

Figure 4.10   X-ray showing a broken neck of femur. The pelvis is to the right and part of the head of the femur remains in the cup-shaped socket in the pelvis. The broken end of the femur has shifted outwards, away from its normal alignment. (Source: Robert Destefano/Alamy)

4.3.1 Decisions about the type of treatment

In general, the type of treatment is determined by the position of the fracture. However, there are other considerations that influence the treatments that are chosen.

◆ Can you suggest any other considerations that you think would influence the treatment undertaken in people with fractured hips?

◆ Possible considerations are the age of the person, their medical fitness, and the available resources.

The *age* of the person is significant because prosthetic replacement hips have a limited lifespan: typically 10–15 years, although this technology is improving. In a young active person, a prosthetic head for the femur would wear out and require replacing at regular intervals, whereas in older people, a 10–15-year solution might provide them with mobility for the rest of their life. Interestingly, the blood supply to the hip changes with age (in children there are additional blood supply routes to those shown in Figure 4.9a), which might also influence treatment options.

The *medical fitness* of a person is a measure of the ability to survive the major operation that might be involved in treating the fracture. For example, the presence of serious diseases such as chronic obstructive pulmonary disease (COPD) and heart disease would make major surgery more dangerous.

The *resources* available depend on factors such as the geographical location of the patient and his or her socio-economic situation. Whilst hip repair surgery is commonplace in the most economically developed countries, there are many parts of the world where facilities for such operations are not available. The cost of these procedures will also exclude poorer people in countries without adequate public health-care provision, where the cost of hospital care must be paid for by patients or their families.

◆ ──────────────

'Prosthetic' means an artificial replacement part that can be attached to the body.

4.4 Falls in older people

The implications of trauma can be far reaching and can influence a person's (and sometimes their family's) longevity and quality of life. In many societies, traumatic injury has the greatest consequences for older people and their carers, with major implications for health services and national health expenditure.

Older people might experience trauma in a variety of ways. In addition to the *physical trauma* that results from injury, loss of work and its associated sense of identity might result in *psychological trauma*; single or multiple bereavements might lead to *emotional trauma*, and loss of independence due to deterioration in physical and sensory functioning may be perceived as *social trauma*.

Physical traumatic injury can have catastrophic personal consequences for older people living anywhere in the world, but this section will focus primarily on the implications of falls in older people in developed countries. In Chapter 1, Figure 1.7 showed mortality associated with falling for older people worldwide. UK data reveals that falls are the main cause of death from injury in people over the age of 75 and a major cause of disability in older people. In 1999, there were 647 721 emergency room attendances and 204 424 admissions to hospital for fall-related injuries in the

UK population aged 60 years or over. These falls cost the UK health service £908.9 million of which 63% related to people aged 75 years and over' (NICE, 2004).

In the USA, after cardiovascular disease, cancer, stroke and pulmonary disorders, 'unintentional injuries' are the most frequent cause of death in older people. Falls cause substantial rates of both mortality and morbidity; 40% of people over the age of 65 living at home fall at least once a year, resulting in 1 in 40 being admitted to hospital. Although most falls don't result in serious injury, about 5% involve either a fracture or a hospital admission (Rubenstein, 2006). Older people living in institutions have higher rates of falls than those living in their own homes, and also higher rates of fractures or lacerations. Falls often result in mobility problems and in western societies may force older people to move from their homes into nursing or residential care (choices of alternative care are not usually available in developing countries).

NICE is the National Institute for Health and Clinical Excellence in the UK. It is an independent organisation responsible for providing guidance on promoting good health and preventing and treating ill health.

4.4.1 Why do older people fall?

◆ What do you think are the main factors that cause falls in older people?

◆ *External* factors: uneven surfaces, poor lighting, poor design of housing, lack of handrails, uneven stairs; *poor physical health*: sight and hearing deficits, balance impairment, muscle weakness or gait (way of walking) problems; *poor mental health*: confusion, cognitive (processing and understanding) and memory difficulties, inappropriate doses of medication.

Table 4.1 shows that accidents and external factors are the most common cause of falls.

Table 4.1 Causes of falls in elderly adults in the USA: summary of 12 studies that evaluated elderly persons after a fall and specified a 'most likely' cause. (Source: adapted from Rubenstein, 2006, p. ii38)

Cause	Mean percentage	Range/%*
'accident'/environment-related	31	1–53
gait/balance disorders or weakness	17	4–39
dizziness/vertigo	13	0–30
drop attack	9	0–52
confusion	5	0–14
postural hypotension	3	0–24
visual disorder	2	0–5
fainting	0.3	0–3
other specified causes (arthritis, acute illness, drugs, alcohol, pain, epilepsy and falling from bed)	15	2–39
Unknown	5	0–21

Drop attacks are sudden spontaneous falls followed by swift recovery.

Postural hypotension is a fall in blood pressure that occurs when changing position (from lying to sitting or from sitting to standing).

*The range is the lowest and highest percentage of falls attributed to this cause in the 12 studies.

Although most falls in older people are *accidental,* they occur because age and disease interact with environmental dangers. Causes applicable to younger people, such as alcohol or substance abuse, may also precipitate falls in older people. But, because older people's bodies tend to be more inflexible and less well coordinated, 'Posture control, body orienting reflexes, muscle strength and tone and height of stepping all decline with ageing and impair ability to avoid a fall after an unexpected trip or slip' (Rubenstein, 2006). How people fall may determine the types of injury. Falling backwards or forwards onto the hand can lead to a wrist fracture; hip fractures usually occur when falling sideways, whilst falling onto one's bottom usually doesn't result in broken bones (Rubenstein, 2006). Fractures differ between age groups: people aged 65–75 are more likely to break wrists, whilst those over 75 more often break their hips, probably because slower reflexes prevent them from protecting themselves with outstretched hands.

Walking requires joint mobility, appropriate timing and intensity of muscle action, and normal responses to visual and sound cues. In a study of people over 75, 10% needed help crossing a room, 20% needed help to climb a flight of stairs, and 40% could not walk half a mile. 'Gait problems can stem from simple age-related changes in gait and balance as well as from specific dysfunctions of the nervous, muscular, skeletal, cardiovascular and respiratory systems or from simple deconditioning following a period of inactivity' (Rubenstein, 2006).

◆ Dizziness is another common cause of falls; what might cause this?

◆ Dizziness is caused by a variety of factors including medication, depression, and cardiovascular disorders.

The *'mental'* state of older people may be linked to falling. A California study exploring osteoporotic fractures in older women found that depressed women fell more frequently than those who were not depressed (Whooley et al., 1999). Older women with more disturbed sleeping patterns (i.e. they take more frequent naps during the day) are at greater risk of falling and developing fractures (Stone et al., 2006). However, it cannot be assumed that either depression or disturbed sleep are the *cause* of the falls in studies such as these; there are too many other factors in people's lives that could make them more likely to fall *and* more likely to become depressed or sleepless. Epidemiologists refer to these as confounding factors.

As many older people have multiple medical conditions (e.g. anaemia and acute illness), it is more relevant to identify *risk factors* rather than attempt to disentangle the causes of individual falls.

Most falls occur in older people's homes and they, as well as relatives and carers, express concern about safety alone at home. Older people in developing countries face similar problems but most do not have access to technological advances available in western societies such as 'call-out necklaces' which are worn around the neck and can be used to transmit a signal to alert carers in the event of an emergency.

◆ What are the problems that might face an older person returning home after being admitted to hospital following a fall?

◆ Returning 'home' following a fracture (or even elective surgery for hip replacement) can be fraught with difficulties, both short- and long-term. Remaining in even a modified home may be problematic and the benefits (familiarity of surroundings both within and outside the home) must outweigh the risks. Many western homes are hazardous, with loose rugs, telephone and electrical wires and rickety furniture. Factors to be evaluated include lighting, bath and toilet facilities, stair banisters, and bed types. Fractures or even serious bruising as a result of falls affects basic physical functioning, including access to and within the home using a Zimmer frame or wheelchair, cooking and personal care. Additional factors to be considered include access to shops, medical facilities, transport and social interaction.

For older people following a fall or other accidental trauma, coping with long-term disabilities resembles coping with impairments such as arthritis, respiratory disorders and visual difficulties. These can lead to older people neglecting their health, poor nutrition, isolation, depression, confusion and other mental impairments. It is not therefore surprising that approximately 40% of all people admitted to residential and nursing homes in the UK have sustained a fall prior to admission.

In summary, older people have a high susceptibility to injury because they are more likely to have complex medical problems, such as osteoporosis, as well as having slower reflexes due to their age. Although children and younger people may fall more frequently, falling is more likely to cause damage in older people. They are likely to recover less quickly, and may experience 'post-fall anxiety' where the person reduces normal activities in order to avoid falling; this can lead to weakness, abnormal gait and paradoxically therefore an increased risk of falling.

4.4.2   Strategies to reduce the incidence of falls in older people

In the USA, an analysis of falls resulting in death estimated that 66% were potentially avoidable (Rubenstein, 2006). In 2003, the UK National Health Service (NHS) introduced a nationwide 'falls service' to reduce the number of falls resulting from balance impairment, muscle weakness, excessive or insufficient medication use and environmental hazards. This was an implementation of the National Service Framework for Older People Standard 6: 'to reduce the number of falls which result in serious injury and ensure effective treatment and rehabilitation for those who have fallen'. By 2006, 74% of UK hospital trusts had a designated falls service, which usually included the following:

Case/risk identification – whereby older people who have reported falls or are seen to be at risk of falling are assessed to ascertain whether they could benefit from interventions to improve their balance and mobility.

Multifactorial falls risk assessment. This might include: assessment of gait, balance and mobility and muscle weakness; assessment of osteoporosis risk; assessment of the older person's perceived functional ability and fear relating to falling; assessment of urinary incontinence; assessment of cognitive impairment and neurological examination; assessment of visual impairment; assessment of home hazards; cardiovascular examination; and medication review.

Multifactorial interventions. These might include: strength and balance training; home hazard assessment and intervention; vision assessment and referral; medication review with modification/withdrawal.

Falls prevention. Encouraging the participation of older people (and carers) in falls prevention programmes including education and information giving.

(Adapted from NICE, 2004)

Falls services also aim to expedite rapid responses to falls, increase capacity in osteoporosis services, scan for bone density (a measure of bone strength) as a guide to treatment, and improve rehabilitation services for people who have impaired functional ability or have lost confidence following a fall (Department of Health, 2006). Similarly, falls prevention strategies have been introduced in other countries. For example, in New Zealand (La Grow et al., 2006) home safety programmes delivered by occupational therapists reduced falls significantly amongst visually impaired older adults.

Falls prevention services include household adaptations and exercise as well as education programmes. Exercise programmes can improve body mechanics, endurance and strength, (Rubenstein, 2006) but only have a limited effect on those with cognitive impairments (Hauer et al., 2006).

In order to understand why some prevention programmes are successful and others are not, older people's views about fall prevention programmes were sought in six European countries (Yardley et al., 2006). Respondents aged 68–97 reported being encouraged to participate by family as well as health practitioners. They believed that strength and balance training provided benefits in addition to fall prevention: for example, interest, enjoyment, improved health, mood enhancement and increased independence. Their negative views about training related to denying their risk of falling, a belief that training in falls prevention was unnecessary, a dislike of group activities, and practical barriers to attendance, e.g. transport, cost and effort.

Now try Activity 4.1.

Activity 4.1   Falls in older people

Allow about 30 minutes

Now would be a good time to go to the DVD associated with this book and watch the short film entitled 'Falls in older people'. This contains two interviews with women who have experienced falls and are describing their experiences. They have both attended an exercise rehabilitation class in South London for older people who have had falls, which is run by a therapist who they refer to as Patrick. The second interviewer suffers from spinal problems which affect her mobility and increase the risk of falling. She mentions receiving injections for pain relief including an 'epidural' which involves injection of medication next to the spinal cord within the spinal canal, and 'facet' injections which deliver medication into the joints between the vertebrae of the spine.

Question 4.7 at the end of this chapter is based on the accounts in these interviews, so you may wish to read it before you watch the video and make notes to help you construct your answer.

Summary of Chapter 4

4.1   Damage to tissues is investigated in many ways including taking X-ray images to visualise fractured bones, and checking for nerve damage or blood vessel damage. Fractures are classified according to the type of damage to the bone (e.g. greenstick) and whether the overlying skin is broken.

4.2   Fractures are treated by realigning the broken bones (sometimes using surgery) and holding them in place while they repair. This can be done using splints, casts, traction and fixation devices. Infection control is an important part of effective treatment.

4.3   The exact location of a hip fracture is important because in some positions a fracture will damage the blood supply to the head of the femur. Broken hips may be repaired or replaced depending on the location of the fracture and the patient's age, medical fitness and resources available.

4.4   Older people have a higher susceptibility to falls-related injury because they are more likely to have complex medical problems, and slower reflexes.

Learning outcomes for Chapter 4

After studying this chapter and its associated activities, you should be able to:

LO 4.1   Define and use in context, or recognise definitions and applications of, each of the terms printed in **bold** in the text. (Questions 4.1 and 4.5)

LO 4.2   Describe what each test (X-ray, nerve function, arterial pulse) detects following traumatic injury. (Question 4.2)

LO 4.3   Describe the main types of fracture in terms of how they might occur (e.g. to a particular age group, following particular types of accident) and how they are identified (by X-ray and visual inspection). (Questions 4.1 and 4.5)

LO 4.4   Discuss the likely impact of availability of care on survival and recovery rates in a global context. (Questions 4.3 and 4.4)

LO 4.5   Describe the factors that are taken into consideration when deciding which treatment to use following a hip fracture (e.g. the position of the fracture in relation to the blood supply, the age and health of the patient and the resources available). (Question 4.4)

LO 4.6   Describe the common causes of falls in older people and discuss strategies to reduce the incidence of these falls. (Questions 4.6 and 4.7)

Self-assessment questions for Chapter 4

Question 4.1 (LOs 4.1 and 4.3)

Figure 4.11 is a diagram of an injury to the bone in a person's upper arm. What type of injury is this, and what particular risk is associated with this kind of damage?

Question 4.2 (LO 4.2)

Describe some tests that would be undertaken in hospital when assessing a patient with a fractured limb.

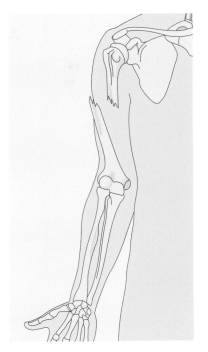

Figure 4.11   Fracture of the arm.

Question 4.3 (LO 4.4)

Traumatic injuries such as those shown in Figures 4.11 and 4.12 could potentially occur to people anywhere in the world, but the seriousness of the outcome and level of survival and recovery vary enormously. Briefly explain the main reason for this variation, assuming that there are no immediate life-threatening problems such as severe blood loss.

Question 4.4 (LOs 4.4 and 4.5)

Hip fractures can occur as a result of various incidents including traffic accidents, sporting injuries, and falls in older people. Describe the main factors that would influence the choice of treatment that might be given for a hip fracture.

Question 4.5 (LOs 4.1 and 4.3)

Figure 4.12 shows some X-ray images of typical fractures. For each one, classify the type of fracture. Briefly describe how fractures are treated in order to allow bones to repair.

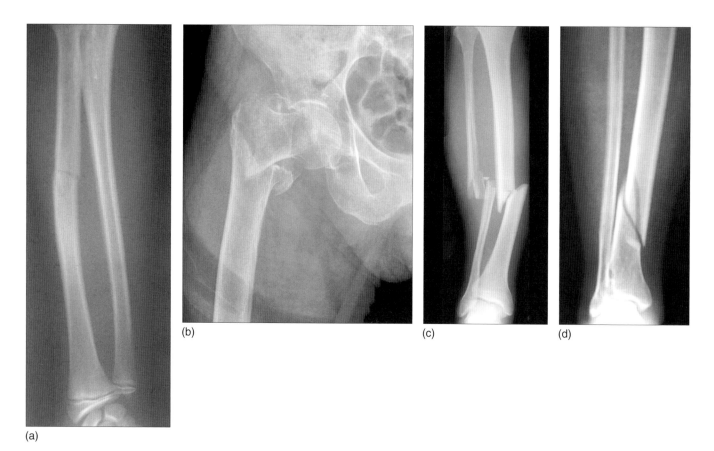

(a)

(b)

(c)

(d)

Figure 4.12 X-ray images showing fractures. (a) A young child's arm after falling from a tree. (Source: © Robert Destefano/Alamy). (b) The hip of a 63-year-old woman with osteoporosis. (Source: Learning Radiology.com). (c) A motorcyclist's lower leg after a collision in which the bone protruded through the skin. (Source: © Medical-on-Line/ Alamy). (d) A fracture to one of the bones in the lower leg of a person involved in a car accident – there was only a slight reddening of the skin to suggest the prescence of underlying damage. (Source: © Phototake Inc./Alamy)

Question 4.6 (LO 4.6)

At the age of 79, May tripped over a suitcase that she didn't notice on a busy station platform, and broke her hip in the fall. Surgical repair and recovery took many weeks before she returned home to her first-floor flat. Some physiotherapy sessions were offered to her, but she was anxious about going out and would only attend if a relative could take her. As time passed she became almost completely housebound, as her confidence waned after several more falls in the house.

What features of May's story may have contributed to her falls?

Question 4.7 (LO 4.6)

DVD Activity 4.1 presented two accounts from women who have experienced falls and have subsequently had to adjust their lives to cope with limited mobility and the fear of more falls. From the interviews, pick out any similarities between the two women's accounts; in particular, what effects have the exercise classes had?

CHAPTER 5

TISSUE REPAIR

5.1 Introduction

In Chapter 3, the leg was used as an example of a part of the body where a number of different tissues interact in order to carry out a function. In Chapter 4 you saw some of the science behind how damage can affect certain tissues – in particular, bone – and the kinds of treatments that are carried out.

This chapter will build on the previous sections and will explore the *repair* that takes place following traumatic injury. The repair characteristics of the tissues you met in Chapter 3 will be discussed in order to give an insight into the processes that occur simultaneously in the different tissues following an injury.

The title of this chapter is 'tissue repair'. The word **repair** suggests that something is being mended, and that the finished product will always 'have been repaired' rather than be the same as when it was new, i.e. regenerated (Box 5.1). This is easy to understand in the context of manufactured objects such as a car, a house or a vase – the repaired version may be 'as good as new' in that it regains its functional characteristics, but it is never the same as an object that was never damaged in the first place. In biology, this is also often the case – at some stage most people have suffered some kind of trauma which has created a wound on their skin. Whilst in most cases these heal quickly and the barrier function of the skin is restored, a scar is left behind and that area of skin will never look quite the same as it did before the damage (Figure 5.1). Skin repair and scarring will be discussed in more detail later in this chapter, but the point to be made here is that a repair usually does not return the tissue to its pre-injury state – tissues tend to repair with scarring.

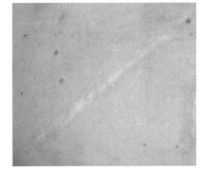

Figure 5.1 A scar where damaged skin has repaired. (Source: Erik Walbeehm)

Box 5.1 (Explanation) Repair or regeneration?

The human body tends to *repair* following damage – mechanisms exist for mending the tissues so that function is restored, however, repaired tissue tends to take the form of a scar. Some organisms are able to *regenerate* tissues following damage. Regeneration suggests that the tissue is 'recreated' rather than repaired. True regeneration can occur in mammalian fetuses at certain stages of development, and can also be seen in some amphibians that have a mechanism for regenerating entire limbs following damage. At the end of this chapter, we will discuss some of the current research in 'regenerative medicine' the goal of which is to regenerate human tissues following damage.

Whilst clinical interventions such as those discussed in Chapter 4 can make a big difference to how well a patient recovers from a traumatic injury, repair depends largely on the natural processes that take place within the tissues. For example, an orthopaedic surgeon can realign a fractured bone and pin it in place, or straighten a greenstick fracture and immobilise the area in a cast, but the final outcome depends on the ability of tissues to repair themselves following damage.

As you work through this chapter, you might like to check back to Chapter 3 to remind yourself about the structure of each of the tissues. At the end of this chapter, you should work through the animation sequences in DVD Activity 5.1 which will reinforce what you have learned about tissue repair. This chapter starts with skin repair because people tend to be most familiar with skin injuries.

5.2   Skin repair

The great majority of traumatic injuries involve skin damage, and many more minor injuries involve *only* skin damage. One of the main functions of the skin is as a barrier to protect the underlying tissues. The skin therefore possesses repair mechanisms focused on the rapid restoration of this barrier function.

The sequence of events following skin damage is well understood because, unlike internal tissues, skin can be monitored very easily during repair. First, blood from damaged blood vessels in the skin fills the wound area and starts to clot. Certain proteins dissolved in the blood respond to damage by becoming insoluble (i.e. they are no longer able to stay dissolved in the blood so they separate out of solution). These proteins then form a mesh of fibres (a clot) that functions like a temporary extracellular matrix. Instead of being made from the usual extracellular matrix proteins like collagen, these structures are made from the protein *fibrin*. **Fibrin** is the insoluble fibrous protein that makes the dense mesh clot; when it is in its soluble form (circulating dissolved in the blood under non-injury conditions) it is called *fibrinogen* (i.e. the material that *gen*erates fibrin).

◈   What do you think is the main function of the dense fibrin clot that forms following skin damage?

◆   To act as a temporary barrier, rapidly restoring the barrier function of the skin.

In addition to clot formation, an inflammatory response follows skin injury. During **inflammation**, fluid collects in the damaged area causing swelling, redness (the redness is due to increased blood flow around the area which is also why inflamed skin feels hot) and pain.

Within a few hours, the fibrin clot dries to form a scab giving temporary protection to the underlying damaged area, which starts to repair. The repair involves stimulation of cells in the dermis (look back at Figure 3.18) called **fibroblasts** that play a key role in the repair of many tissues because they can migrate into wound sites and make new extracellular matrix proteins such as collagen (Figure 5.2).

◈   What new structural feature do you think enables fibroblasts to migrate into the wound area?

◆   The fibrin clot.

The fibrin clot forms a temporary extracellular matrix which the fibroblasts populate, and then replace with collagen. As well as laying down new collagen, the fibroblasts contract and pull the sides of the wounded dermis together. At the same time, epidermal cells divide and migrate to cover the healing dermis, creating a thin layer of new epidermis within about 48 hours. Over the next week or so, this grows

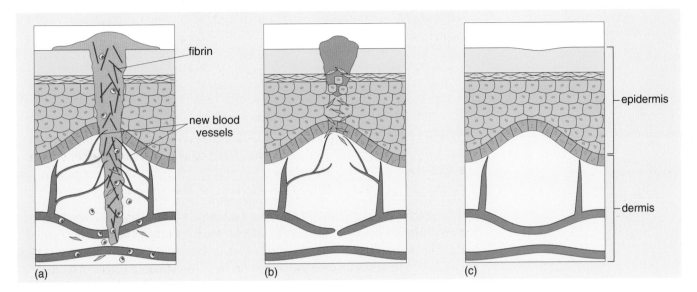

Figure 5.2 Skin repair. (a) The fibrin clot becomes infiltrated with blood vessels and fibroblasts from the dermis and is gradually replaced with new extracellular matrix proteins such as collagen. (b) Other cells from the epidermis and dermis invade the area. (c) Eventually the granulation tissue disappears and the newly healed skin takes on the characteristic layered appearance.

to become the multilayered epidermis of normal skin (Figure 3.18). The new tissue at the site of a repairing skin wound is called **granulation tissue** because it has a number of tiny newly formed blood vessels that give it a grainy appearance.

The next stage in skin repair is that many of these tiny blood vessels (which formed to aid the initial repair process and having done so then become superfluous) disappear, returning the grainy red skin to its normal colour. The new collagen fibres are remodelled to resemble the normal architecture in the dermis and the epidermis takes on the characteristic layered appearance.

◆ In your experience, does healed skin look exactly like normal skin?

◆ It depends on the extent of damage. After minor damage, healed skin can be restored to its previous appearance. After more extensive damage (deeper wounds or larger areas affected), healed skin takes on a scarred appearance.

Scars form where tissue healing has taken place and they are not quite the same in structure as the original tissue. For example, scarred skin often lacks features such as hairs and sweat glands. It also tends to have a less organised structure of collagen fibres. This is because normal collagen architecture gradually forms in response to mechanical forces generated during movement and growth. These are largely absent in the healing wound and as a result new collagen is laid down in a random orientation. Scar tissue is therefore not as strong and durable as normal tissue and is sensitive to further damage. Scars take time to form and the process by which scarring occurs is known as **fibrosis** in which the fibroblasts which formed the temporary granulation tissue go on to produce large amounts of more permanent collagen fibres. Serious scarring of skin not only looks unsightly, but can lead to difficulties in function. In particular, contraction of large scars can restrict movement (Figure 5.3).

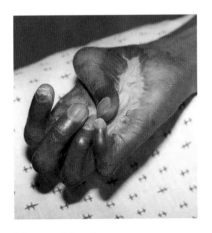

Figure 5.3 Severe scar contraction. (Source: Mercy Ships UK)

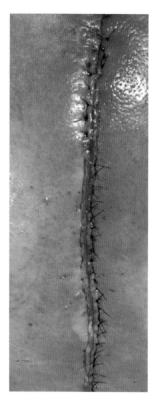

Figure 5.4 Sutures holding the sides of a skin wound together in order to allow it to heal. (Source: Erik Walbeehm)

◆ Look at Figure 5.3. What do you think makes a large area of scarring contract like this?

◆ A scar contains fibroblasts that have the ability to contract (they pull the sides of skin wounds together during normal healing), so lots of fibroblasts in a large scar will result in a lot of contraction.

Before skin wounds can heal, they need to *close*: the sides of the wound need to be brought together. In larger wounds, or those in places where the skin is under a lot of tension, it is often necessary to hold the wound closed using *sutures* (Figure 5.4).

In very large skin wounds, or where disease interferes with healing, sometimes it is necessary to graft skin onto the damaged area. In such cases, layers of skin can be peeled from other parts of the patient's body and used to repair damaged areas. The normal repair processes then enable the donor site to repair itself, and the grafted skin becomes integrated into the skin surrounding the wound site.

5.3 Bone repair

With its highly specialised mineralised extracellular matrix and capacity to withstand heavy loads and large forces, bone might appear to be one of the more difficult tissues to repair. From a biological point of view, however, bone has a remarkable capacity for repairing itself. As discussed in Chapter 3, bone is a living tissue containing cells that continuously form bone (osteoblasts) and these are balanced by cells that continuously resorb bone (osteoclasts).

◆ What function does this system of constant production and resorption serve?

◆ This process means that there is a constant turnover of bone tissue, which enables it to respond to changes in demand (for example, as the body grows bones can get longer).

This inherent capacity (known as *remodelling*) is what gives bone the ability to repair so well following damage. Once a fracture has healed, the normal osteoclast and osteoblast activity will remodel the healed region until it is almost indistinguishable from undamaged bone. During remodelling, the collagen that forms fibres and gives the bone tissue strength gets moved around until it is positioned in the optimal orientation. A good analogy would be to consider a rope: the strength comes from the organised manner in which the rope fibres are laid down – a jumble of fibres that were not carefully twisted together would have little strength. During repair, the bone extracellular matrix fibres are produced in a random orientation, but then during remodelling they are gradually reorganised to become strong support structures.

So, a healed bone fracture can be remodelled to resemble undamaged bone, but how does the fracture heal in the first place?

When a bone breaks, blood leaks out and fills the area of damage. At this stage, it is possible to realign the broken parts of the bone by manipulation (if they are displaced), but eventually this blood starts to clot to form a fibrin scaffold for the repair processes that follow. One of the important cell types that migrates into this scaffold are the **stem cells** which naturally reside in bones. Stem cells are special cells that can divide to produce 'daughter' cells that can become a selection of different cell types. The stem cells that migrate into the bone injury site can divide to give rise to new osteoblasts. These new osteoblasts populate the damaged area and start to make new bone.

◆ What two things must the osteoblasts do in order for bone to be formed?

◆ Osteoblasts secrete collagen and organise the mineralisation of the extracellular matrix (see Section 3.3.1).

◆ In order for the newly formed osteoblasts to survive, what needs to be present at the site of repair?

◆ A blood supply, bringing oxygen and nutrients.

One of the most important events that occurs early on in this process is that the clot (more accurately known as a *callus* once the osteoblasts start turning it into bone) becomes *vascularised* (vas-cue-lah-rized); this means that a network of capillaries is assembled throughout the scaffold that then supplies the repair cells with oxygen and nutrients. These capillaries grow into the repair site from nearby undamaged tissue.

This repair stage can take many months, and is then followed by the remodelling stage where the newly produced bone extracellular matrix is gradually organised into the correct shape for optimal function.

The stages in the bone repair process are summarised in Figure 5.5 and can be followed by viewing the animations in DVD Activity 5.1. We suggest you work through the next few sections on how other tissues repair, including Box 5.2, then turn to Activity 5.1 and watch the repair sequences.

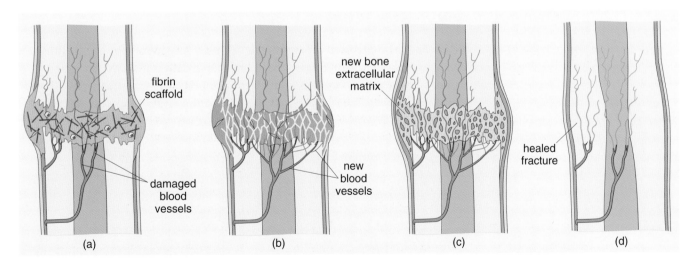

Figure 5.5 Stages in bone repair. (a) Damage to the blood vessels at the fracture site causes leakage of blood which clots and forms a fibrin scaffold that supports the migration of stem cells and new osteoblasts into the repair site. (b) New blood vessels develop and the temporary fibrin scaffold is replaced with collagen. (c) Gradually the fibrin scaffold is completely replaced with bone extracellular matrix molecules and becomes mineralised. (d) The new bone extracellular matrix eventually remodels to become strong supporting bone.

Box 5.2 (Enrichment) A little more detail on how bones repair

When new osteoblasts are formed at the damage site, they detect the level of oxygen and nutrients in their local environment and this influences their fate. If there is a good supply of oxygen and nutrients, as happens once the callus has been thoroughly vascularised, then bone production proceeds as described above. If the blood supply is poor, as it often is near the middle of the repair site, then instead of becoming osteoblasts the cells turn into the kinds of cells that are normally found in cartilage, and in fact the tissue at this site of repair resembles cartilage rather than bone. With time, this cartilage-like callus is invaded by capillaries and more osteoblasts and eventually gets replaced by bone.

◆ What is the main difference between bone and cartilage?

◆ Cartilage does not have the mineral components that make bone hard (Section 3.3.1).

The description of bone repair in this section should make it clear why the clinical interventions discussed in Chapter 4 are useful for helping fractures repair. Rather than interfere with the natural healing process, the medical staff realign and immobilise the damaged bone in order to give it the best chance of healing itself.

◆ Why is it important to realign and immobilise a fracture?

◆ To hold the damaged pieces of bone in position so that the repair process is not disrupted by movement and so the broken ends knit together in the correct position.

As well as holding the broken parts together to facilitate repair, casts and other stiff devices which are used to immobilise bone are effectively taking over the mechanical support role that the damaged bone normally fulfils as part of the musculoskeletal system. It is important to remove the stiff supporting cast as soon as possible after sufficient repair has occurred in order to expose the newly healed bone to some (gentle) mechanical forces so that the remodelling phase can occur.

Whilst the availability of modern healthcare clearly makes a big difference to people who have had traumatic injuries, especially in terms of initial life support (Chapter 2), pain control and reducing infection risks (Chapter 4), it is interesting to note that as far as treating fractures is concerned, the fundamental approach of providing a stiff support has not changed since ancient times. Archaeological investigations of Egyptian mummies have revealed the treatment of fractures using splints made of wood, reeds or bamboo. The intrinsic ability of bone to repair itself means that there is little else that can be done except immobilise and let nature take its course.

5.4 Muscle repair

Muscle can be damaged by traumatic injury in a number of ways: in particular, by being cut, torn or crushed (Box 5.3). Small tears and 'pulled' muscles are frequent occurrences during over-exertion and these heal rapidly, so it is clear that there are effective intrinsic repair processes in this tissue.

Muscle tissue is very rich in blood vessels; in fact, the fluid content of muscle tissue is so high that it is estimated that 80% of the water in the body resides in the muscles.

Muscle damage inevitably results in damage to the blood vessels and bleeding within the muscle. Initial damage results in inflammation during which fluid collects in the damaged area causing swelling and pain.

Box 5.3 (Enrichment) Crush injuries

Myofibres contain chemicals that, whilst essential for muscle function, can be harmful if they are released into the blood circulation. During severe crush injuries this can be a serious problem. Crushed muscles sustain a high degree of damage to their myofibres, which release these toxic chemicals. This can be made worse during sustained crush injuries because the blood supply can be cut off, resulting in more damage, and more inflammation causing fluid release into the area (which, in turn, can cause swelling, increasing the local pressure and making the damage worse). When the crushing force is removed and circulation is restored to the damaged muscle, the blood supply to the rest of the body becomes flooded with the harmful chemicals. This can result in damage to organs such as the kidneys.

Initial inflammation following muscle damage can be reduced by gently compressing the muscle (e.g. in a bandage) and elevating it (i.e. raising the foot or hand).

◆ Why might elevation of a limb with a damaged muscle help reduce inflammation? (Think back to Chapter 2.)

◆ Elevation will encourage blood flow back towards the heart due to the effects of gravity, helping to relieve the build-up of fluid at the site of injury.

The repair process following muscle damage depends on the extent of the injury. The healing response that follows initial inflammation involves the formation of a temporary fibrin scaffold, similar to the situation discussed above with regard to skin and bone repair. This temporary scaffold gradually becomes populated with a network of capillaries and fibroblasts that make extracellular matrix proteins, forming granulation tissue (Figure 5.6).

In minor injuries to muscles, the granulation tissue provides a scaffold for myofibres to grow through and bridge the damaged area. In more extensive injuries, the granulation tissue is not fully replaced by new muscle, and fibrosis leads to the formation of scar tissue instead.

Repair occurs through the fusion of myoblasts to myofibres. The process is similar to the mechanism by which the myofibres form during muscle growth (Section 3.3.2 explained that myo*blasts* merge together to make long single myo*fibres*, each of which has many cell nuclei). In order for this to occur, there must be a supply of new myoblasts to repair the damaged muscle tissue. New myoblasts are formed by the division of stem cells residing in the muscles, which respond to the chemical signals produced at the site of damage. The stem cells can divide rapidly and produce a large number of new myoblasts which can fuse with damaged myofibres and facilitate muscle repair. Repair is followed by a period of remodelling, during which the new tissue is gradually orientated into its characteristic alignment.

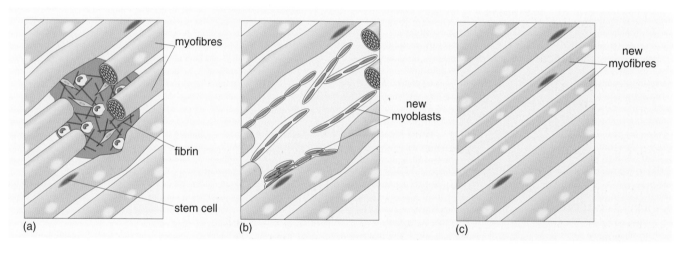

(a) (b) (c)

Figure 5.6 Stages in muscle damage and repair. (a) The initial damage to the muscle results in the formation of a fibrin scaffold that becomes populated with capillaries and fibroblasts. There are stem cells in the muscles. (b) The stem cells multiply to produce new myoblasts that can fuse with damaged myofibres to repair them (bottom of b), or can merge together to form new myofibres to replace those that have been badly damaged (middle of b). (c) Finally the new and repaired myofibres at the repair site become fully integrated into the muscle and the temporary fibrin scaffold is completely replaced by collagen and other extracellular matrix molecules.

5.5 Tendon repair

So far this chapter has discussed tissues with a good inherent capacity for repair (skin, bone and muscle), but when tendons are damaged they do not repair themselves very well.

◆ Consider the structure of tendon tissue (Section 3.3.3) and suggest a feature that might be responsible for poor healing.

◆ Tendons have a poor blood supply compared with muscles and bones. This means that the supply of oxygen and nutrients is limited, thus limiting the number of cells that can be present. Since cells are necessary for removing debris and building new tissue, tendons are therefore disadvantaged when it comes to repair.

Given the limited number of cells and lack of blood vessels in tendons, one might ask the question: 'How do tendons manage to become such dense and effective tissues in the first place; surely lots of cells are needed to produce and remodel all of that extracellular matrix protein?' In fact, during development when tendons are forming they are richly populated with cells and have a good blood supply. As they mature, the cell population dwindles and the blood supply is reduced to the minimum level required to support the small population of cells responsible for maintenance.

Because of the low self-repair ability, surgical interventions are common when a tendon is damaged. Sometimes, if a tendon is cut or torn, it is possible for a surgeon to stitch the ends back together; this provides structural integrity and restores the function of the tendon.

◆ What is the function of a tendon?

◆ It connects a muscle to a bone and conducts force from one to the other; so as a muscle contracts, the bone moves.

If a large area of a tendon is damaged, which is possible when trauma affects the tendon directly, then there may be insufficient tendon tissue remaining for the surgeon to stitch the damaged parts back together. In such cases, a graft can be used. A graft is where some undamaged tissue is used to replace tissue that has been damaged. The undamaged tissue can come from a less critical part of the body (often a small strip of tissue harvested from a neighbouring tendon), or be taken from another person. When a graft comes from the same person it is called an **autograft** (*auto-* means 'self') and when it comes from another person it is called an **allograft** (*allo-* means 'other'). Note that allografts are frequently obtained from dead people, and 'tissue banks' exist in many countries as a repository where donated tissue is stored prior to use. One of the problems with allografts is that tissue that the body does not recognise as being its own can cause an immune response during which the donor tissue may be 'rejected'.

The terms 'autograft' and 'allograft' are generic and can be used to refer to all types of tissue (e.g. skin autografts), not just tendon.

Because tendons and ligaments have a similar structure (Section 3.3.3), they are sometimes used interchangeably for grafting repairs.

◆ What is the most important feature of the tissue that is used for a tendon graft?

◆ The graft tissue will have the highly organised and strong extracellular matrix structure that is required to withstand force and restore function.

The big challenge when it comes to grafting tendons is attaching them firmly to the bones. Sometimes this problem is overcome by harvesting the donor tendon with part of the bone still attached (i.e. the surgeon cuts through the donor bone, leaving the tendon/bone interface intact), then using the bony end of the tendon to anchor it in its new position.

◆ What would be the advantage of repairing a tendon with a graft that still has a piece of bone attached?

◆ The new attachment would be bone to bone rather than tendon to bone, so would exploit the good healing properties of bone to achieve the repair.

Some repair processes do take place in damaged tendons following surgical interventions. These processes are similar to those already described in other tissues: the damaged area becomes inflamed and a fibrin scaffold forms, then fibroblasts lay down new collagen, forming temporary granulation tissue which is gradually replaced with permanent collagen and other extracellular matrix proteins (Figure 5.7). With time and gentle mechanical loading, the new collagen can become aligned and strong, and tendon function can be restored. However, whilst the weight-bearing properties of the tendon are restored through the

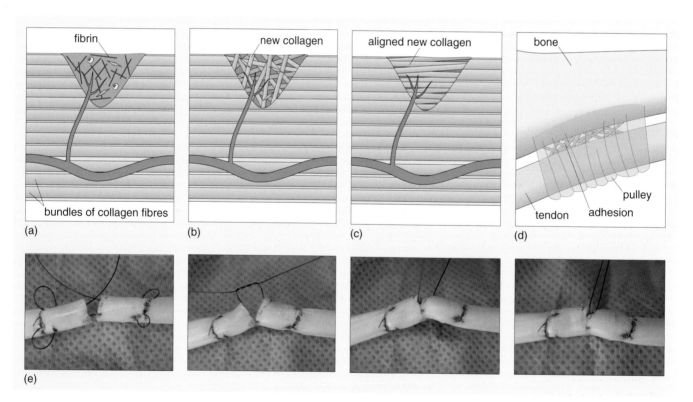

Figure 5.7 Repair in tendons. (a) A fibrin scaffold supports the ingrowth of tiny capillaries and fibroblasts. (b) The fibrin is gradually replaced with collagen. This process can take a long time because the blood supply in tendons is relatively poor compared with other tissues. (c) Eventually the collagen is remodelled to become strong and aligned. (d) In some cases the production of collagen at the site of damage can make an adhesion form between the tendon and surrounding tissue. (e) Tendon surgery uses strong sutures to hold the severed ends of the tendon together and protect the repair site from load. (Photo: Erik Walbeehm)

synthesis and remodelling of collagen, the elastic fibres are not restored so the tendon will not be as elastic under heavy load as it once was.

Fibrosis and the formation of scar tissue can cause particular difficulties during repair of tendons. Fibroblasts deposit collagen in random orientations and sometimes in the wrong places.

◆ Can you think of a bad place for new collagen to be deposited in a repairing tendon?

◆ Tendons need to move over their surrounding tissues, especially where they run through pulleys and sheaths (Section 3.3.3). If new collagen is laid down between the tendon and the surrounding tissue, then the tendon will stick instead of moving freely.

This **adhesion** (Figure 5.7d) of tendons to their surroundings, caused by fibrosis, is a major problem when it comes to tendon surgery. In a clinical setting, the tendon needs to be immobilised in order for the best repair to take place between the severed ends, but immobilisation means that there is an opportunity for adhesion with the surrounding tissue. These factors both need to be taken into account to optimise recovery.

5.6 Nerve repair

Because of their key role in sensation and muscle control, damage to peripheral nerves can cause widespread problems. A loss of sensation in the hand or foot can effectively mean a loss of function. Without being able to feel pressure through the hands and feet, many tasks would be impossible. Without feeling pain, serious tissue damage from further trauma becomes inevitable. If the nerve connection between the CNS and a muscle is damaged, then the muscle cannot contract and will deteriorate. As is the case for tendons, nerve injuries do not heal easily (whereas bone, skin and muscle have a relatively good capacity for healing to a level where function is restored, albeit with scarring).

Damaged *peripheral* nerves can sometimes repair to some extent, but the *CNS* has little capacity for repair. Spend a few minutes reminding yourself about nerve structure (Section 3.3.4).

◆ Neurons are the cells responsible for the conduction of action potentials. If a traumatic injury cut through a peripheral nerve half way along a limb, which parts of the neurons would be damaged?

◆ The injury described would cut through the axons of all of the neurons. The peripheral nerves that run along the limbs are bundles of axons supported by Schwann cells and extracellular matrix structures (Section 3.3.4).

The reason that peripheral nerves can sometimes repair following this type of injury (where one part of the nerve is cut or crushed by trauma) is that damage to the axon of a neuron, even completely cutting through it, does not always kill the whole neuron. The axon is a long thin projection leading away from the cell body. Cutting through a peripheral nerve means that the part of the axon that has been detached from the cell body disintegrates, but the part that remains attached to the cell body (containing the nucleus) can sometimes survive (Figure 5.8a).

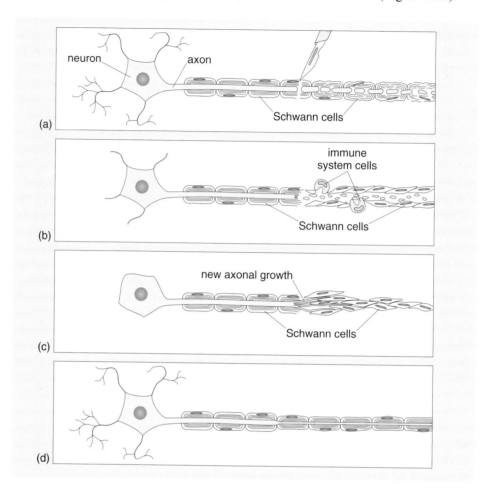

Figure 5.8 Peripheral nerve damage and repair. (a) If an injury cuts through an axon then the part of the axon that has been detached from the cell body disintegrates, (b) The debris is cleared away by other cells. (c) The Schwann cells that were surrounding the part of the axon that disintegrated now form a pathway that can guide axonal re-growth from the end of the remaining axon. (d) Eventually this process can result in growth of the axon all the way to the target and a restoration of function.

The surviving part of the axon may be able to extend again, guided by the other structures in the nerve such as the Schwann cells and the meshwork of collagen fibres that remain intact beyond the injury site. This means that if the severed ends of a cut nerve are sutured back together, then it is possible for the surviving axons to elongate back down the paths left behind when the previous cut-off parts of the axons disintegrated (Figure 5.8c). When axons finally reach their target (for example a muscle or part of the skin), then some function may be restored.

However, there are three main problems with nerve repair.

The first relates to the time it takes for neurons to regrow: axons elongate at approximately 1 mm per day.

◆ How long would it take for restoration of a nerve connection to the foot following damage to the sciatic nerve in the thigh?

◆ This depends on the length of the leg; but, for example, if this distance was 60 cm, then assuming a growth rate of 1 mm a day it would take 600 days (about 20 months).

The problem is that during this time, with no stimulation while waiting for motor neurons to re-grow, the unused muscle would deteriorate. If sensory neurons were cut then there would be an area with no sensation until the axons re-grew. This part of the body would be highly susceptible to further damage during this period.

The second problem is the size of the gap. If the nerve is cut, rejoining the stumps in the manner described can be achieved by a skilled surgeon. However, traumatic injury often damages a large section of the nerve, leaving a gap. Axons will still grow out, but if a gap is present there will be little to guide them across it. Growth at 1 mm a day is not much use if it is not in the right direction. Furthermore, if axons do not find the appropriate route then they might form synapses with tissue surrounding the repair site which can have painful consequences. Because of these problems, nerve grafts are often used: surgeons can remove part of a less important nerve and use this as a bridge to join the two nerve stumps across a gap. Because removing part of a nerve to make a nerve graft involves cutting through the axons and separating them from the rest of their neurons (in particular the cell body which contains the nucleus), the axons in the piece of donor nerve will not survive.

◆ What would a nerve graft supply in this situation (since it does not contain living axons)?

◆ It would supply a scaffold for guiding and supporting repair, made from the extracellular matrix proteins and the Schwann cells in the donor nerve.

The third problem is adhesion. As in other tissue repair situations, fibrosis takes place at sites of nerve damage and the collagen that is produced can sometimes stick the nerve to the surrounding tissue.

◆ What problems might be caused by adhesions between a nerve running through the leg and its surrounding muscle tissue?

◆ Peripheral nerves need to be able to move independently of the surrounding tissue, slipping over muscles that are contracting and bending and stretching around joints. If adhesions form, parts of the nerve will be anchored to the surrounding tissue and tension pulling on the nerve could result in nerve damage or pain during movement.

5.7   Blood vessels

It should be apparent from reading the descriptions above of how different tissues repair, that blood vessels play a pivotal role. The growth of new capillaries into a site of repair is an important feature which accompanies other natural repair processes.

◆ What do you think is the main purpose of rapidly building a capillary network at the site of a repair?

◆ Repair involves division, migration and action by cells, which need a source of oxygen and nutrients from the blood in order to survive and carry out their function.

This process of building new blood vessels is known as *angiogenesis* (*angio* (an-jee-oh) is derived from the Greek for a vessel, *genesis* refers to generation) and involves the branching and extending of the existing capillary network. In response to chemical signals, endothelial cells lining existing vessels become active, dividing to make more cells and modifying their extracellular matrix so that they are able to sprout new branches of vessels into the new tissue.

Traumatic damage to large vessels poses a serious threat to the cardiovascular system, as discussed in Chapter 2. Once blood loss has been controlled, it is sometimes necessary to carry out surgery to repair damaged blood vessels if they are large and important. A surgeon may be able to suture the cut edges of vessels back together. Grafts of blood vessels are also used in many cases, enabling important vessels such as those that supply the muscle of the heart with blood to be replaced by less important vessels from elsewhere in the body (a coronary artery by-pass operation).

Now try Activity 5.1.

Activity 5.1   The repair of tissues in the leg

Allow about 1 hour

Now would be the ideal time to turn to Activity 5.1, a multimedia exercise on the DVD associated with this book which returns you to the material you studied in Activity 3.1 (the three-dimensional arrangement of tissues in the leg). This time you will focus on the repair sequences that take place in each of the tissues. If you cannot study this activity now, do so as soon as possible; it will reinforce what you have learned about the repair processes in the major tissues in the leg.

5.8   General repair issues

The previous sections discussed the differences and similarities in the ways in which different tissues heal. No two traumatic injuries are identical, and it is likely that a whole range of tissues will be injured to different extents. The initial treatment (Chapter 2) to stabilise the patient and reduce life-threatening issues is universal, but the treatment that follows and optimises tissue repair and recovery of function depends on a wide variety of factors.

◆ Name the different tissues that might be injured in one single traumatic injury. As an example, consider the mid-thigh injury sustained by Hassan as a result of his motorcycle accident (Vignette 4.1).

◆ The main tissues likely to be injured are bone, muscle, blood vessels, nerve, tendon and skin.

Most tissues benefit from immobilisation in the early stages of repair to enable the fragile temporary extracellular matrix structures to become replaced with more robust tissue. However, remodelling and strengthening of the repaired tissue in response to mechanical forces produced by movement is also often required. This is fine if only one tissue is injured (it can be immobilised for the appropriate length of time and afterwards gently exercised), but if a fast-healing tissue such as skin or muscle is kept immobilised for a long time to enable a slower healing or more damaged tissue (bone, nerve, etc.) to achieve better repair, then the fast-healing tissue may suffer.

◈ What other problem might be exacerbated by long periods of limb immobilisation?

◆ Adhesions. This is a problem with tissues such as nerves and tendons whose function can be impaired by the formation of adhesions with the surrounding tissue.

A rehabilitation programme of gentle movement may help to reduce the formation of adhesions, but this might be detrimental to the healing of other tissues involved.

The purpose of this chapter is to explore the complexity of multi-tissue injuries that result from trauma. Whilst the mechanisms of tissue repair, and the most appropriate clinical interventions to optimise outcome, are well understood, in reality any treatment is likely to be a compromise between the best approaches for each of the tissues involved. As with all clinical interventions, treatment will also depend heavily on the facilities available in terms of specialist healthcare provision, the speed with which treatment can be provided, and the range of long-term follow-up therapies available for rehabilitation and care.

In addition to differences in the extent of injury and the availability of treatment options, there is wide variation in how well individuals recover from traumatic injury.

◈ Can you think of any factors, other than extent of injury and quality of care, which might influence how well a person recovers?

◆ Age is an important variable in recovery from injury, as is the overall health of the person, their psychological state and their level of expectation.

5.8.1 Age

All tissues change with age and these changes can be very dependent on the life experience of the individual. For example, the skin of a person who has been routinely exposed to high levels of sunlight is likely to be more wrinkled and less elastic than that of someone the same age who was not exposed to the same high levels of sunlight. This is a complex area of research, made more so by the difficulties faced by researchers in trying to separate the effects of age from those of life experiences, and a detailed discussion is beyond the scope of this book. However, when it comes to bones, there is a consensus that they generally become weaker with increasing age.

◈ Do you remember from Section 3.3.1 what happens to bone during the lifespan of a person?

◆ During childhood and early adulthood, the balance between formation and resorption of bone favours formation; from middle age onwards, this balance shifts towards resorption.

In many people, this poses no problem at all: their bones are sufficiently well-formed at middle age that even the inevitable resorption of bone tissue during their remaining years does not result in sufficient weakness to undermine function. However, because of this change in balance between formation and resorption under normal conditions in bone, healing of fractures is inevitably less robust in later life.

5.8.2   Health

There are a great many disease states that can affect the extent of damage and the effectiveness of tissue repair. Surviving a traumatic injury, and subsequent repair of tissues places a severe burden on the body's resources. Anything that compromises the body's ability to cope with this burden is likely to reduce the chance of a successful outcome.

◆   What processes occur during repair that might increase the demands placed on the body?

◆   Tissue repair involves increased cell division, increased cellular activity (e.g. migration and matrix remodelling) and increased production of tissue components (e.g. proteins such as collagen).

These processes increase the demand for energy and for the production of molecules involved in repair. If health is damaged by infection or disease, then the body will not be able to meet this extra demand and repair will be impaired. In people who are malnourished, tissue repair will be less successful than if they were provided with a diet rich in foods that supply energy, protein and vitamins (Box 5.4).

Box 5.4 (Enrichment) Vitamin C

Collagen production by cells involves the assembly of amino acids (the individual building blocks of proteins) into large fibres that provide structural support for the tissues. This assembly process requires the chemical commonly known as vitamin C (ascorbic acid). Insufficient vitamin C in the diet causes *scurvy*, which results in damage to tissues where collagen turnover is high (in particular, the extracellular matrix of blood vessels and the fibres that hold teeth in their sockets resulting in bleeding and loss of teeth). Increased collagen production is necessary for tissue repair, so lack of vitamin C will reduce the effectiveness of repair after trauma.

5.8.3   Expectation

So far, we have discussed tissue repair with regard to achieving restoration of function. However, the success of repair is a very difficult concept to measure. It relates to the individual's expectations, previous life experiences, and future plans (living with disability will be discussed further in Chapter 6). It is useful at this stage to flag up the observation that evaluating the extent to which tissue repair has been successful is partly subjective, as Vignette 5.1 demonstrates. Read through the vignette, then think of your own examples of people who might receive identical injuries, with identical outcomes in terms of tissue repair, but would differ in how they might describe the level of functionality of the outcome.

Vignette 5.1   Evaluating the outcome of repair (Tony and Teresa)

Tony is a professional footballer who plays in one of the top UK teams. He has two young sons and one of his favourite ways to relax when off the pitch and away from the public gaze is to kick a football around with them in the large park opposite their house. One evening, Tony puts his left hand out to stop a tumble during an enthusiastic tackle, and cuts it on some broken glass that is hidden in the long grass at the edge of the pitch. When he looks more closely, he realises that the wound is quite deep and there is a lot of blood, so he goes to hospital to have it checked. On examination, the medical staff realise that as well as a deep wound, Tony's little and ring finger are numb and he can't feel any pressure when they touch the skin on those fingers. The glass has cut through one of the nerves in Tony's hand. Surgeons are able to suture the ends of the cut nerve back together and within a few months some sensation has returned to the fingers. This part of Tony's hand is never quite the same again, but within a few weeks he is back on the football pitch and continues to play for the rest of his career at the top of his profession.

Teresa is a classical pianist, the same age as Tony, and at the peak of her profession. She has travelled all over the world and played in front of many audiences. When she is not travelling, she enjoys relaxing with friends and after one dinner party at a friend's house she insists on helping with the washing up. She plunges her hand into the soapy water and realises too late that there is a sharp knife submerged beneath the bubbles. She receives an almost identical injury to the one Tony received from the broken glass, and the nerve is repaired by the same surgeon. After a few months, there is some sensation restored to the finger tips, and the function that returns is equivalent to Tony's. However, the function never returns the hand to the same state as before the injury, and Teresa cannot play the piano at a professional level again.

5.8.4   The future of tissue repair

Even with the most advanced clinical approaches, there are limitations to the effectiveness of tissue repair. Fundamental to this is the concept discussed at the outset of the chapter (Box 5.1) – the difference between repair and regeneration.

Currently the very best outcome for tissue repair tends to be a tissue with restored functionality, but that is not as good as the tissue was before the damage. For example, repaired skin might be an excellent barrier, but it may look different to normal undamaged skin and be more susceptible to damage. There are also problems with large wounds where tissue may need to be replaced by grafts. Tissue elsewhere in the body that can be harvested for autografts is limited and creates a second site of damage. Donor tissue for allografts also has limited availability and may cause immune reactions if the body does not recognise the tissue as being its own.

In recent years, there has been a huge research effort in this area with the aim of overcoming some of these problems. This has led to the emergence of **tissue engineering** which, as the name suggests, involves building replacement tissues in order to restore function.

◆ What are the main constituents that would need to be included in an engineered tissue?

◆ Tissues are mixtures of cells and extracellular matrix with the appropriate mechanical properties for function. You might also have thought of the need for a blood capillary network.

Research in this field has used a variety of approaches, which tend to involve building some kind of support scaffold (to mimic the extracellular matrix), then seeding it with the appropriate cells. The idea is that this can be implanted into the wound, where it will integrate with the host tissue and aid repair (Figure 5.9). There are many issues that need to be considered: the scaffold materials used need to be compatible with the body, have the right mechanical properties, and eventually be replaced by natural extracellular matrix. Scaffolds can be made from natural extracellular matrix proteins or synthetic materials. The cells need to be obtained from somewhere (cell populations can be expanded in laboratories, enabling a small number of cells harvested from a patient to be expanded into sufficient numbers for a repair) and they need to be given the appropriate environment to encourage repair processes.

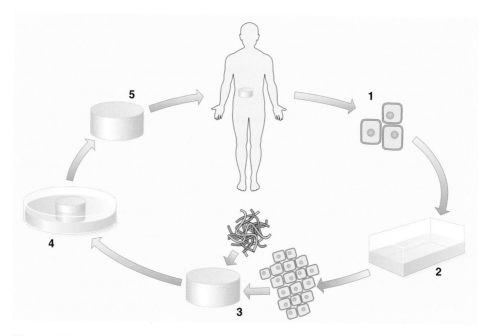

Figure 5.9 Typical tissue engineering approach: (1) remove cells; (2) expand number of cells; (3) seed cells into scaffold and (4) allow 'engineered' tissue to develop; (5) implant engineered tissue into repair site.

Some tissue-engineered products have been used successfully in the clinic and many more are likely to follow. The future for tissue engineering is likely to be targeted towards *regeneration* rather than repair. This exciting area, often called **regenerative medicine**, takes the concept of engineering tissues beyond aiding repair and on to building new tissues in a similar manner to the way in which they form naturally (rather than the way they repair). A key advance in this field is the use of stem cells to provide a source of cells required for building tissues. Earlier in this chapter, the stem cells that normally reside in the body were mentioned due to their involvement in supplying new cells for repairing bone and muscle. Stem cells can divide to produce new cells that can become a selection of cell types with different specialised functions (Figure 5.10).

◆ Name some cell types you have learned about in this book.

◆ Osteoblasts (Section 3.3.1), osteoclasts (Section 3.3.1), myoblasts (Section 3.3.2), fibroblasts (Section 5.2), neurons (Section 3.3.4), Schwann cells (Section 3.3.4), keratinocytes (Section 3.3.5), epithelial cells (Section 3.3.5), endothelial cells (Section 3.3.6).

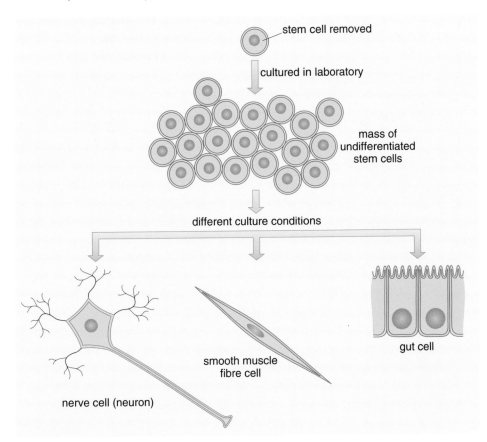

Figure 5.10 Stem cells can divide to make more stem cells and to become a selection of different cell types.

Specialised cells all have particular names because they are different to each other structurally and they each serve a specific function. They can be identified by the way they behave or by the molecules they make. If they divide, the daughter cells are identical to the parent cell. These properties make these cells *differentiated*, i.e. they have adopted a particular identity. Stem cells are not like this – they are not differentiated. They can divide to give rise to daughter cells that can develop into a variety of different types of differentiated cells. This means that a stem cell is a very powerful resource for regenerative medicine; stem cells grown in a laboratory could theoretically be used as an endless source for any type of cell in the body (since they continuously replenish themselves).

The idea of using stem cells for therapeutic purposes is not new; indeed, bone marrow transplants have been used for treating patients with leukaemia for many years (bone marrow is a source of stem cells which can differentiate to replace the white cells that are affected in leukaemia). However, concerns about the long-term fate of cells implanted into the body, the use of human embryos for research and therapy, and the difficulties in maintaining and controlling stem cells, are all issues that need to be tackled before the potential of these new approaches can be realised.

In theory, harnessing the power of stem cells would enable a truly regenerative approach to tissue healing: replacement tissues could be grown from scratch in the laboratory or at the site of a repair. In practice, there is much yet to be learned about how to obtain, maintain and control stem cells, and the development of this technology has provoked much debate about the ethics of the approach.

If you are studying this book as part of an Open University course you should now turn to Activity C2 in the *Companion*.

Summary of Chapter 5

5.1   Tissues that are damaged by trauma tend to repair with scarring due to fibrosis which produces randomly organised extracellular matrix.

5.2   The sequence of events that occurs in tissues follows a general pattern: formation of a fibrin clot, then infiltration of the fibrin scaffold with cells and blood vessels (formation of granulation tissue), then replacement of granulation tissue with new tissue or scar tissue.

5.3   Different tissues heal at different rates with different levels of success. Bone takes a long time to heal but the inherent remodelling that occurs in normal bone (due to the activity of osteoblasts and osteoclasts) means that repair is normally very successful. Muscle and skin are also very effectively repaired but often with scarring.

5.4   Tissue healing depends largely on the presence of cells that can replace the temporary fibrin scaffold with more appropriate extracellular matrix, and the presence of a blood supply to nourish these cells. Stem cells are an important source of new cells at the site of repair. Tissues with few cells (e.g. tendons) repair poorly compared to other tissues.

5.5   Peripheral nerves can sometimes repair following damage to the neurons, but this depends on the ability of axons to re-grow from the area above the damage all the way to the target area of the body. If a gap is present, then a graft can be used.

5.6   Fibrosis following damage can sometimes result in adhesion between tissues that would normally be separate.

5.7   Repair following major tissue damage depends on the extent of the damage and the health, age and psychological state of the patient as well as the availability of specialist treatment and rehabilitation.

5.8   Current advances in tissue engineering and regenerative medicine aim to repair and regenerate tissues using technology such as artificial scaffolds and stem cells.

Learning outcomes for Chapter 5

After studying this chapter and its associated activities, you should be able to:

LO 5.1   Define and use in context, or recognise definitions and applications of, each of the terms printed in **bold** in the text. (Questions 5.1, 5.2 and 5.3)

LO 5.2   Briefly describe the general repair mechanisms that tissues undergo following damage. (Question 5.1)

LO 5.3   Describe the mechanisms and extent of recovery from injury of the six named tissues. (Question 5.2)

LO 5.4   Describe the concept of 'regenerative' medicine and summarise some of the benefits and issues associated with research in this area. (Question 5.3)

If you are studying this book as part of an Open University course, you should also be able to:

LO 5.5   Describe how a journal article is organised and discuss how the intended audience for a piece of writing will determine its content and style. (Activity C2 in the *Companion*)

Self-assessment questions for Chapter 5

Question 5.1 (LOs 5.1 and 5.2)

Fibrin, which forms a fibrous mesh during blood clotting, is often referred to as a 'temporary extracellular matrix'. Explain why.

Question 5.2 (LOs 5.1 and 5.3)

Many different tissues can be damaged during a traumatic injury, but some repair more successfully than others. Compare and contrast the healing properties of bones with those of tendons and comment on the likely degree of functionality of the outcomes.

Question 5.3 (LOs 5.1 and 5.4)

Briefly describe what a stem cell does during normal repair. Stem cells are considered to be useful for the future of regenerative medicine. What advantages might stem cell therapies have over autograft and allograft approaches?

LONG-TERM PERSPECTIVES

This final chapter takes a step back from examining the details of tissue damage and repair and considers some of the long-term consequences of trauma. In the first section the lasting psychological damage that occurs in some people will be discussed, then the cost of trauma to individuals, families and societies in different parts of the world will be considered.

6.1 Long-term psychological consequences

You read in Chapter 1 that road traffic accidents are a major cause of physical trauma: they are also a serious cause of psychological harm (Figure 6.1). It is easy to appreciate that suffering physical injuries is liable to be psychologically damaging, for example as a result of the pain and anxiety. What may be more surprising is that, even in circumstances where the accident leaves a person physically unscathed, serious psychological damage may result. This is illustrated in DVD Activity 6.1 which includes an interview with a woman who survived a bomb attack on a London Underground train but suffered psychological damage as a result. It is also explored in Vignette 6.1.

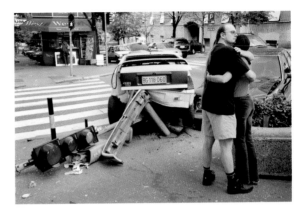

Figure 6.1 Passengers comfort each other after being involved in a car accident in which one vehicle crashed into a set of traffic lights near a zebra crossing in Belgrade, Serbia. (Source: Martin Roemers/Panos Pictures)

Vignette 6.1   Dave's story

Dave was involved in an accident on a motorway, when an articulated lorry crossed the central reservation into his lane. His car was crushed almost out of recognition, and he was pinned inside for a long time before the rescue teams were able to cut him free. When he was finally extracted and checked over by the ambulance crew it was found that, miraculously, he had escaped with nothing worse than cuts and bruises. But while he was trapped in the tangled wreckage, with the growing smell of petrol, he really thought he was going to die; his passenger did.

Understandably, Dave was very shaken by his experience; he found it hard not to keep thinking about it, and his sleep was badly affected. Two months later, when things were, if anything, worse, he went for professional help. He told the psychologist that he had nightmares, and during the day he'd suddenly 'see' the scene and 'smell' the petrol, almost as if it were happening all over again. As he described this, the psychologist noticed that Dave gradually contorted himself in his chair, apparently adopting the position into which he had been forced in his mangled car. Dave said that he had tried a little driving since the accident, but he couldn't face a motorway – even watching articulated lorries from a motorway bridge filled him with a sense of panic. He couldn't get fuel for his car, because the smell of petrol immediately brought on the horrible *flashbacks* (i.e. feeling vividly that he was part of the event once more). His concentration was poor, and he felt tired and irritable all the time.

The story of Dave, in one form or another, is all too common. Similar kinds of aftermath can be experienced by people caught up in major disasters, or women who have been raped, and also by military personnel after exposure to horrific scenes. Dave's friends congratulated him on having escaped such a terrible crash with hardly a scratch. However, from his perspective there was little to be congratulated about; his life was in ruins. He couldn't do his job properly, and he had lost interest in everything that he used to enjoy, from a drink with friends in the pub, to making love with his wife. He had all the classic symptoms of **post-traumatic stress disorder (PTSD)**.

The defining features of this condition are listed in an internationally used manual referred to as DSM IV, which is the **D**iagnostic and **S**tatistical **M**anual of Mental Disorders, fourth edition (IV is a Roman four). DSM IV lists an enormous range of mental conditions from which people can suffer, and sometimes the distinctions between the conditions are quite subtle. So that clinicians and researchers across the world can communicate, knowing that they are talking about exactly the same condition, it is important to have a manual that makes it possible to define precisely how each condition is to be diagnosed. So, what does DSM IV have to say about PTSD?

6.1.1   What is PTSD?

To be classed as PTSD, the unpleasant symptoms must have lasted longer than the usual short-lived response to a very stressful situation: they must be of greater than one month's duration. The manual is also rather precise about the kind of circumstances that initiated the problem. To be PTSD there must have been a distinct precipitating event, in which the sufferer's own life or well-being were seriously threatened, or where someone else at the scene was similarly threatened. Dave had both of these; he was frightened for his own life, and his passenger actually lost hers.

◆ Can you think of a reason why the *legal* system has shaped the definition of PTSD, to require a specific traumatic incident, rather than say a series of very stressful events, which might equally lead to similar symptoms?

◆ Western societies are becoming increasingly litigious (i.e. likely to sue for damages in a court of law) and large awards for damages may await someone who can go to court and claim to be suffering from PTSD. The claim has to be made *against* someone (for example, the lorry driver's insurance company) but to make the accusations 'stick' they cannot be vague claims: there must be a specific time and place, which can be identified as the cause of the condition.

Dave's principal problem is not being able to keep the event out of his mind for very long. Things such as the smell of petrol easily trigger the memory again, and when it comes it has a far more vivid 'here-and-now' feel than ordinary memories. You can probably remember where you went on a holiday or a trip to another town, but it is unlikely that you can conjure up those memories so vividly that you feel you are back there again. Another difference between PTSD memories and normal memories is that the latter do not keep forcing themselves into your consciousness. You can *decide* to recall something from the past, but when you don't wish to, the images do not fill your dreams and interrupt your work. Why would our memory systems have developed in such a way that the misery of PTSD is possible?

◆ The evolutionary history of the ancestors of modern humans involved the accumulation over time of traits (i.e. characteristics) that improved the chances of survival. Living longer gave an individual more opportunity to have offspring and pass on those traits. Why might it be useful from an evolutionary perspective for memories of highly threatening events to be very easily triggered?

◆ An animal that formed easily triggered memories of situations that it had only just survived, would, as a result of the associated fear, be less likely to get into similar situations in the future.

Consequently, the animal would be likely to live longer, and pass on its genes (including those that contributed to this memory process) to more offspring. They, in turn, would be more likely to survive longer and reproduce than the offspring of animals lacking this trait.

Our ordinary memories, for things such as holidays, meetings, changing jobs and so on, comprise what is known by psychologists as **autobiographical memory**. They form a rich tapestry that almost defines who we are, rather as a portrait captures something of a person. These are all 'well-behaved' memories; some may not be happy, but even then they don't keep intruding, unbidden, into our conscious thoughts. Researchers in the field of PTSD (e.g. Ehlers and Clark, 2000; Conway and Pleydell-Pearce, 2000) are agreed that memories for traumatic events are not stored in autobiographical memory in the same way; somehow, trauma memories stand out from other events, in frightening relief. Conway and Pleydell-Pearce suggested that trauma memories fail to be integrated into autobiographical memory, because they are a threat to our ordered self-view, which is based upon the normal contents of our autobiographical memory. To protect the existing sense of self, the storage system tries to exclude the new, unpleasant material. As a result, the memories sit obtrusively in a kind of no-man's land. This account goes some way to explaining at a descriptive level what might be going on, but it makes no attempt to explain the underlying biological processes. To understand these, we need to consider some of the brain structures that are probably involved. Chief among the brain regions implicated in PTSD are the *hippocampus* and the *amygdala*. Their locations in the brain are shown in Figure 6.2.

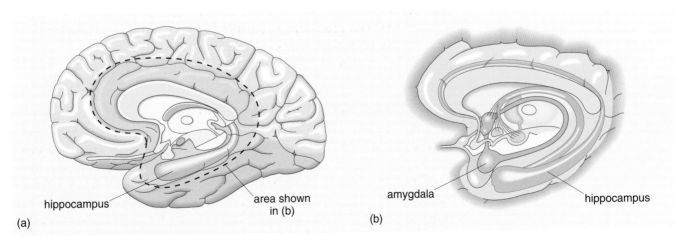

(a) hippocampus   area shown in (b)   (b) amygdala   hippocampus

Figure 6.2 A vertical slice through the centre of a brain. (The front of the brain is to the left.) (a) Position of the hippocampus. (b) An enlargement of the area within the dotted line in (a).

6.1.2 The brain and PTSD

The **hippocampus** is a long, curved structure (shaped rather like a sea-horse, from which its Latin name derives) buried deep within the brain. It contains many neurons, with extensive connections to other regions of the brain. The hippocampus has an essential role in the storage and retrieval of memories. London taxi drivers are required to learn the whereabouts of all the streets listed in the London A to Z (a street atlas of the city); they call this prodigious feat, gaining 'the knowledge'. Brain-scanning has revealed that acquiring the knowledge actually results in a slight enlargement of part of the hippocampus (Maguire et al., 2000). Conversely, alcoholism is liable to result in degradation of the hippocampus, and the sufferer's memory deteriorates; in extreme cases, *Korsakov syndrome* may result. In this condition, it effectively becomes impossible to acquire new memories. The patient may chat to you about life in the past (old memories are intact), but if you leave, to return ten minutes later, he or she will have no knowledge of the conversation, nor even that you had been there!

Interestingly, in the context of PTSD, prolonged stress (not a single traumatic event) seems to be damaging to the hippocampus, so that it actually shrinks in size (Magariños et al., 1997). It is tempting to explain this as a shrinking through lack of use – the opposite to the situation with taxi drivers – because the hippocampus appears to be less involved in laying down memories of highly emotive (e.g. frightening) events. However, the damage may in fact be more related to the high levels of stress hormones (epinephrine and cortisol) circulating in the bloodstream. Nevertheless, the hippocampus does seem to have a lesser part to play in storing stressful material: instead, it is the amygdala that has a key role (Rauch et al., 2000). The **amygdala** is a bean-sized mass of neurons, situated near to the head of the hippocampus (this arrangement is duplicated in each hemisphere of the brain). The amygdalae (plural of amygdala) are known to be involved in processing emotional material, and part of this action may be to modify the way in which the hippocampus stores memories.

As you perhaps guessed from the use of words such as 'seem', 'may' and 'appears to', these processes are still not fully understood. However, a clue as to what may be going on is to be found in the fact that, most of the time, none of the vast number of things we remember enters our consciousness. You are not bombarded with thoughts of trips from home, your name and address (and those of all your friends), your first day at work, teachers at school, etc. What stops the parts of the brain that hold all those memories from making us aware of them at any and every moment? Almost certainly, the activity of the neurons involved is *inhibited* by the frontal areas of the brain (an area called the prefrontal cortex). This region is involved in inhibiting many aspects of brain activity. It is not fully developed in childhood, and it also tends to degenerate in old age.

◆ What effects might be expected if the prefrontal cortex is not fully functional in these age groups?

◆ An absence of control from the region would explain why children, and some older people, can occasionally be embarrassingly uninhibited!

So what has the amygdala to do with PTSD? For some reason, memories that have been stored under the influence of the amygdala are far less amenable to inhibition. There are numerous connections between the amygdala and the prefrontal cortex, so the amygdala may be able to act on the prefrontal areas so as to reduce their usual inhibitory activity (Figure 6.3). That leaves the memories liable to pop into consciousness with the least provocation, and a PTSD sufferer is forced to try to avoid anything that might trigger the flashbacks.

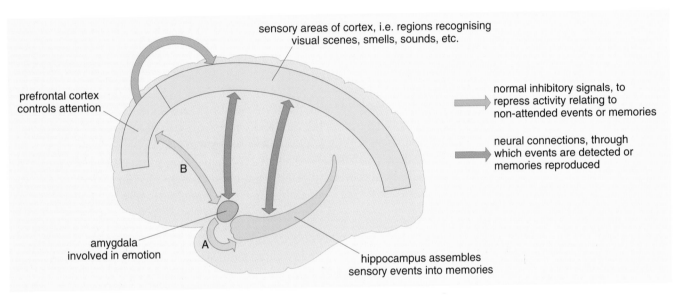

Figure 6.3 A schematic representation of brain regions involved in memory and attention (this slice through the brain has the same orientation as Figure 6.2). The neural pathways, A and B, are known to exist. It is believed that when the amygdala is involved in forming traumatic memories, it modifies hippocampal involvement via pathway A. It is speculated that it also inhibits the attentive processes of the prefrontal cortex, via pathway B, so making it difficult to keep emotional material 'out of mind'.

We will end this section on a more cheerful note, and consider what happened to Dave (Vignette 6.2 overleaf).

Vignette 6.2   Dave's treatment

The first step in Dave's treatment was to work on his feelings of guilt. He knew, logically, that the accident was not his fault, but he had felt guilty for living, when his passenger had died. This is a common element of PTSD; soldiers will feel guilty for surviving when comrades have died, and perhaps more remarkably, women who have been raped sometimes experience feelings of guilt for being attacked. While an affected person maintains a strong sense of guilt, it can be difficult to alleviate the symptoms of PTSD; it is almost as if he or she feels that their unhappiness is in some way deserved. To alleviate the guilt, the psychologist spent time getting Dave to talk about the feeling, then challenging him gently, whenever his reasoning was illogical. Little by little, Dave's intellectual recognition that, in theory, he had nothing to feel guilty about was broadened, so that he really *felt* that he was not guilty. The psychologist instructed Dave that, when he was at home, or out and about, without his psychologist to talk to, he should adopt the therapist role, and challenge *himself* any time he felt himself slipping back into the feelings of guilt. The psychologist's method of helping, simply through conversation and instruction, is sometimes referred to as a 'talking therapy'.

With the guilt issue in hand, the prime goal of Dave's therapy was to get the terrible events on the motorway to form a part of his everyday autobiographical memory system. It would always be an unpleasant memory, but it would nevertheless be relegated to the position of 'just another memory'. That would be achieved by getting him to go through the story several times, remembering it vividly, but at the same time remaining calm.

◆ What might take place in Dave's brain, if he rehearsed a previously frightening event, while in a more calm state of mind?

◆ With the fear element reduced, his hippocampus would be able to regain its usual role in laying down a memory of the event. With less involvement from the amygdalae, the memory would be amenable to inhibition from the prefrontal cortex.

Although not an essential technique for treating PTSD, the psychologist decided to use hypnosis with Dave. Hypnosis is a state of mind that is usually induced in a person by getting them to shut their eyes and relax. A susceptible person easily responds to suggestions, for example that they do not feel pain. Dentists have used this technique instead of anaesthetics. There have been a number of reports that hypnosis is a valuable adjunct to the treatment of PTSD (e.g. Carter, 2005). Sufferers tend to be more responsive to hypnosis than the average member of the population. Why this should be so is not known; it may be that enhanced hypnotic susceptibility is brought on by the trauma, but alternatively being susceptible to hypnosis in the first place may make people more vulnerable to PTSD, if they are unlucky enough to experience a major trauma. It has been suggested by Bryant et al. (2003) that the first explanation may be the right one.

Whatever the explanation, Dave responded well, so first of all he was helped to experience a very calm, safe feeling. From this firm foundation,

Chapter 6 Long-term perspectives

the psychologist then moved on to what therapists sometimes call the video technique. Dave had to imagine himself watching a video of the events on the motorway; in hypnosis, this kind of imagining can be as vivid as the real thing. He had the imaginary video controller, so was able to stop the images if he wished, fast-forward, go back – whatever he liked. In this way, not only could Dave gradually get used to the scenes, but also, seeing them as if on a TV meant that he was no longer feeling as involved. It was almost as if the man in the car was someone who just happened to look like him. When he was fully at ease with watching himself being cut out of the wreckage, the psychologist asked him if he was ready, in hypnosis, to enter the picture and be that man. He agreed, and before long was describing the experience calmly.

◆ In a research study (Felmingham et al., 2007), PTSD patients were shown anxiety-provoking pictures, first before, then after they had been treated. What changes might you expect in the way their brains responded to the pictures after treatment?

◆ Brain scanning showed that, after the patients were treated, the pictures evoked *more* activity in a frontal brain region and *less* in the two amygdalae.

Six months after his treatment was complete Dave returned for a follow-up appointment. He was able to report that he had made several motorway journeys and, apart from wincing at the price, had no trouble in filling his fuel tank!

Dave's story, like many of the vignettes in this book, is designed to give you some insight into the profound effects that trauma can have on people's lives. Section 6.2 explores the cost of trauma in a global context, but first Activity 6.1 will provide an insight into what it is like to live with the long-term effects of having experienced serious trauma.

Activity 6.1   Life after trauma

Allow about 30 minutes

Now would be a good time to go to the DVD associated with this book and view Activity 6.1 which explores the experiences of two individuals who are living with the aftermath of trauma. Their accounts are highly personal and emotive and some people may find them upsetting. The interviewees are a man who was involved in a motorcycle accident and received multiple injuries including a head injury and a woman who was involved in a bomb attack on a London Underground train and experienced PTSD.

Question 6.3 at the end of this chapter is based on one of these accounts, so you may wish to read it before you watch the video, and make notes to help you construct your answer.

6.2   The cost of traffic accidents

This book has explored some of the ways in which traumatic injury, particularly as a result of traffic accidents, affects people's bodies and minds. The effects of trauma on people's long-term well-being are often closely associated with their ability to continue to fulfil the roles they previously occupied (for example, in Activity 6.1 the man who had the motorcycle accident was still unable to return to work several years afterwards).

It is clear that not only do traumatic injuries occur with greater incidence in poorer communities, but these communities are also ill equipped with the immediate and long-term healthcare infrastructure that makes a big difference to outcome following trauma. Like most of the topics studied by health scientists, poverty becomes a major factor influencing the likelihood of traumatic injury (e.g. dangerous road traffic systems, unsafe industrial and agricultural workplaces) and the subsequent quality of care (e.g. the availability of skilled emergency services, access to skilled surgical services, access to long-term disability care and psychological treatment services). Since outcomes depend so heavily on economics, this book will finish by taking a look at some of the economic costs of trauma.

The cost of traffic-related trauma to national economies and individual families is colossal.

◆ What factors would need to be taken into account when estimating the financial cost of traffic accidents?

◆ You may have thought of damage to vehicles and infrastructure (e.g. the wall hit by the bus in Figure 1.10); lost economic output from those involved in the crash; medical and other healthcare costs; and the cost of police time, emergency services and legal expenses.

GDP refers to all the wealth generated within a country, so it takes no account of wealth brought in from outside.

The cost of traffic accidents to the UK economy was estimated at over £12 billion in 2000, or around 1.0% of the country's gross domestic product (GDP). In countries such as Bangladesh, India and Pakistan, the cost of each crash is much lower than in the UK because earnings, goods and services have a lower cash value. But the *rate* of traffic accidents is so much higher that they drain a greater percentage of the country's wealth – 1.6% of GDP in Bangladesh, for example (around US$76 million in 2003). Across the whole of the South Asian region, the annual cost of traffic accidents has been estimated at US$25 billion (Rahman, 2004).

It is exceedingly rare for poor families anywhere in the world to have insurance against loss of livelihood due to injury, and life insurance coverage is relatively rare. As Table 6.1 shows, this means that injuries leading to disability or death can tip households into poverty; for example, in urban Bangalore, 71% of households classified as 'non-poor' prior to the traffic accident became 'poor' afterwards.

Table 6.1 Percentage of households in Bangalore and Bangladesh where a fatal or serious traffic-related injury to a family member resulted in the family becoming poor.* (Source: Global Road Safety Partnership, 2004)

Fatal injuries	Urban (%)	Rural (%)	Serious injuries	Urban (%)	Rural (%)
Bangalore	71	53	Bangalore	17	25
Bangladesh	33	49	Bangladesh	21	37

*Internationally accepted definitions of 'poor' and 'non-poor' were used, based on per capita household-income.

6.3   Final word

This book has taken a multidisciplinary approach to exploring some of the science concerned with trauma, repair and recovery. We started by discussing the incidence of death and injury from trauma and how it varies according to age, gender and geographical location. The major cause of these kinds of injuries and deaths are traffic accidents, which are set to rise in developing countries where motor vehicle usage is increasing rapidly. Importantly, the burden of disability and death from trauma disproportionately affects poorer families and poorer countries. This disproportionality also reflects the fact that survival and recovery from traumatic injuries is heavily dependent on the availability of emergency care and subsequent medical treatment.

You have learned about the systems in the body that are so essential to life that damage to them can rapidly result in death if not treated effectively. Examples from the UK emergency services who are highly trained and equipped to respond rapidly in the event of an accident (Activity 2.2a), contrast starkly with the situation in parts of the developing world, in particular in rural areas where emergency care might be days away, or where the cost associated with such care makes it inaccessible. We described the tissues of the body that are likely to be damaged by trauma, and showed how different tissues with different structures are intimately arranged in a functioning limb to enable movement, support and sensation. Differences in the healing of these tissues were explored, along with some of the current and future healthcare interventions that may improve tissue repair. The focus on how fractures are identified, stabilised and supported during repair, again highlights that differences in outcome depend largely on the level of specialist care that is available.

In places we have stepped away from the tissue biology and explored how traumatic injury affects people in a more sociological and psychological sense. In particular, we looked at the problems associated with traumatic injury in older people and how lives can be permanently changed by falls, or just the fear of falling. Other long-term perspectives highlighted how different people manage to cope with trauma, and how in some there may be long-term psychological 'scars' that remain long after the tissues have healed.

Summary of Chapter 6

6.1   Following a life-threatening situation, even though the person may be physically unharmed, there is a possibility that they may suffer post-traumatic stress disorder and suffer from flashbacks – recurring memories of the trauma, which are far more vivid than normal memories.

6.2   Trauma memories may differ from memories for other events, because the amygdala plays a greater role in their storage (normal memories involve the hippocampus).

6.3   Treatment for PTSD normally uses some form of gradual re-exposure to the traumatic events. Re-exposure is believed to enable the events to be stored in the same way as other memories, so that flashbacks are no longer created.

6.4   The economic and social costs of trauma are massive throughout the world, but the burden of disability and death from traffic accidents disproportionately affects poorer countries and poorer families, in terms of both rates of injury and economic impact.

Learning outcomes for Chapter 6

After studying this chapter and its associated activities, you should be able to:

LO 6.1   Define and use in context, or recognise definitions and applications of, each of the terms printed in **bold** in the text. (Question 6.2)

LO 6.2   Discuss some of the possible long-term effects of traumatic injury (PTSD, loss of income, living with disability, etc.) and describe some ways in which people cope with long-term disability. (Questions 6.2 and 6.3)

LO 6.3   Describe the principal symptoms associated with PTSD, the significance of memory processes in its persistence and the principles underlying treatment methods. (Questions 6.2 and 6.3)

LO 6.4   Discuss the differences in people's experience of traumatic injury and recovery that arise as a consequence of differences in the availability of specialist medical care, long-term rehabilitation provision and loss of income due to death or disability in different communities. (Question 6.1)

Self-assessment questions for Chapter 6

Question 6.1 (LO 6.4)

The chances for survival and recovery following a traumatic injury vary depending on the person's access to specialist care, which means that poorer people are disadvantaged. In what other way can traumatic injury have a disproportionately greater effect on poorer people?

Question 6.2 (LOs 6.1 and 6.3)

It has been suggested that the triggering of flashbacks in people with PTSD may be due to traumatic memories being stored differently to normal memories. With this in mind, explain how the hippocampus and amygdala may represent alternative 'filing systems' for memories.

Question 6.3 (LOs 6.2 and 6.3)

You should answer the following on the basis of what you have seen in DVD Activity 6.1.

(a) Jackie, the woman caught up in the London underground bombing, was diagnosed as having PTSD. Give two of her symptoms which would have led to this diagnosis.

(b) Suggest two of Jackie's experiences during the incident that could have been expected to result in her developing PTSD.

(c) What was the principal characteristic of the treatment that helped Jackie to gain greater control of her symptoms.

ANSWERS AND COMMENTS

Question 1.1

Worldwide, males in all age groups are more likely to die from traffic-related injuries than females in the same age group. The gap between the two sexes is quite small at 0–4 years, larger at 5–14 years (males suffered about 50% more deaths than females) and is greatest in the age group 15–29 years, where nearly 250 000 males died in 2002 compared with around 60 000 females. From the age of 30 onwards, a similar number of females died in each group (around 60 000–70 000), but the number of male deaths gradually declined to about 225 000 at age 30–44 years, 160 000 at age 45–59 years, and about 130 000 in males aged over 60 – when the number of deaths was still almost double that among females.

Question 1.2

There are many reasons including: the rapid increase in the number of vehicles on the roads of developing countries; the large numbers of pedestrians – particularly children – who have to walk to work, school, etc. among fast-moving traffic; the large number of multi-occupancy vehicles; the often poor state of repair of roads outside major urban centres and inadequate measures for reducing accidents; large numbers of unsafe vehicles; and little enforcement of injury prevention measures such as wearing seat belts and crash helmets. The rise in traffic accidents is compounded by often inadequate emergency medical services (e.g. ambulances and paramedics) to transport injured people to hospital quickly enough to save their lives.

Question 2.1

Blood is pumped under pressure from the heart into the arteries that carry it to the different parts of the body. The arteries have thick muscular walls to withstand the blood pressure created by the pumping of the heart. The arteries branch and eventually become small capillaries which run throughout the tissues, delivering the oxygen and nutrients required by cells. The capillaries have thin walls which facilitate the diffusion of oxygen out of the blood and into the tissues. The blood vessels that lead away from the capillaries in the tissues and carry blood back to the heart are veins. These have thinner less-muscular walls than arteries because they do not need to withstand pressure from the heart. Instead, blood moves through the veins as they are squashed by the movement of surrounding muscles. The blood moves in one direction only (towards the heart) due to the presence of one-way valves in the veins.

Question 2.2

Blood loss of up to 10% would not be sufficient to compromise the function of the cardiovascular system and would have no obvious effects. As the blood loss reached 20%, the patient's body would attempt to maintain blood pressure by increasing heart rate and constricting blood vessels in the skin. The pulse would be elevated and the person would look pale. There might be some reduction in the oxygen supply to the brain, causing dizziness. As the blood loss approached 30%, the heart rate would be very rapid and the skin very pale and cold. The person would be showing signs of lowered levels of consciousness as oxygen supply to the brain would be reduced. If blood loss approached 40%, then the body would no longer be able to maintain blood pressure and the patient would lapse into unconsciousness as the nervous system became starved of oxygen. The lack of oxygen supply to the essential body systems (the muscle of the heart and the muscles involved in lung function and the parts of the nervous system that control them) would rapidly result in death.

Question 2.3

Constriction of the blood vessels in the skin would result in an increase in blood pressure. This is because there would be less room for the blood to circulate within the blood vessels, so the pressure would increase. Another way in which the body can achieve an increase in blood pressure is for the rate and size of heart contractions to increase.

Question 2.4

Clenching and releasing the calf muscles will squeeze the veins in the legs, helping to move the blood within them back up towards the heart. This increases the flow of blood back to the heart and prevents a reduction in blood flow to the brain that might result if blood accumulated in the legs due to standing still.

Question 3.1

(a) Protection is the main function of the epidermis which is the outer waterproof layer of the skin made predominantly from dead keratinocytes. The epidermis is thicker at sites where most protection is needed, e.g. the palms of the hands and soles of the feet. Pigments in the base layer of the epidermis provide protection from the harmful effects of the sun.

(b) Sensation is provided by the sensory nerve endings that lie in the dermis. They detect pressure or temperature changes and respond by sending action potentials along their axons to the CNS.

(c) Temperature is regulated by a combination of the hairs which sprout from the dermis (which stand up in the cold, thus trapping a layer of warm air next to the skin), the subcutaneous fat which provides a layer of insulation, the presence of blood vessels in the dermis that can dilate to increase blood flow and reduce temperature or constrict to reduce blood flow and consequent heat loss, and sweat (released from sweat glands in the dermis) that evaporates from the surface of the skin to cool the body.

Question 3.2

The stiffness and compressive strength of bones are largely due to the mineral components which are not present in tendons. The contractility of muscles is due to the myofibres, which are not present in tendons.

Question 3.3

(a) Examples of places where tissues must adhere strongly to each other could include any of the attachment points between muscles and tendons, between tendons and bones, and between bones and ligaments.

(b) Examples of places where tissues need to glide past each other could include areas along the length of nerves, muscles, bones and tendons where other tissues are adjacent but not directly attached and where these tissues might need to move past each other during normal flexion and extension.

Question 3.4

Action potentials generated in the CNS would pass down the axons of the motor neurons in the peripheral nerve that leads to the muscle that extends the leg. This muscle, which is located in the front of the thigh, and various other muscles in the body associated with the kicking action, would contract. This is due to the action potentials stimulating the myofibres within the muscles to shorten, causing the muscles to get shorter and thicker. At the same time, the opposite muscles in the antagonistic pair (which cause flexion) relax. The muscle contraction pulls on the tendon which joins the muscles to the bones in the lower leg, causing extension (straightening) of the knee. Tendons have highly aligned collagen fibrils in their extracellular matrix providing tensile strength and transferring the movement generated in the muscle to the bone at the point of attachment. The tendons run past the knee joint and need to be able to glide easily past the adjacent tissues. The force transferred from the muscle via the tendon pulls on the bones which act as levers and swing the lower part of the leg towards the ball. As the foot makes contact with the ball, sensory nerve endings in the dermis of the foot detect the pressure and generate action potentials that travel up the axons of the sensory nerves to the CNS.

Question 3.5

Force × distance on one side of the fulcrum is equal to force × distance on the other side. Therefore, since force (30 N) × distance (60 cm) to the right of the fulcrum is 30 N × 60 cm = 1800 N cm, the force to the left of the fulcrum will be 1800 N cm/2 cm = 900 N (because the distance to the left of the fulcrum is 2 cm). This means that holding a 3 kg weight at arm's length is equivalent to applying a 900 N load directly to the tissues of the shoulder.

Question 4.1

The injury shown in the figure is an *open fracture* which is also *displaced*. Because in an open fracture the skin is broken, there is an increased risk of infection.

Question 4.2

In hospital, an X-ray image of the damaged area would be taken in order to assess the location and severity of the fracture (and whether it was displaced). Damage to other tissues would also be assessed, in particular checking for a pulse at the end of the damaged limb (a check for blood vessel damage) and for sensation (a check for nerve damage).

Question 4.3

The main reason is the availability of expert medical care and facilities. If there is a delay in treating serious injuries such as these, then the risk of severe infection causing further damage or even death is greatly increased.

Question 4.4

The main factors that would influence the choice of treatment for a hip fracture would be the precise position of the fracture and the age, medical fitness of the patient and the resources available. The precise position is important because, for example, if the blood supply to the detached head of the femur is not damaged, then this part of the bone can be reattached (if the blood supply is cut off, then this part will deteriorate). Age is important because the blood supply is different in younger people, and also prostheses which might be used to repair damage have a limited lifespan so their use in a younger person might be unwise due to the need for renewal.

If a person's medical fitness is in doubt, perhaps due to disease or fragility due to old age, then it might be dangerous to subject them to the major surgery involved in hip repair.

The resources available often limit the choices of treatment. Hip repair requires skilled surgeons and expensive hospital facilities of the kind that are not available to all people who require them.

Question 4.5

(a) Greenstick fracture; (b) insufficiency fracture; (c) open fracture, also displaced; (d) closed fracture, also undisplaced (although some realignment may be necessary in this case). Fractures are realigned, then immobilised using devices such as casts, splints, traction and various fixation devices that might be internal or external.

Question 4.6

Deteriorating eyesight or concentration may have contributed to the original fall in a busy unfamiliar environment. May's age may have been associated with osteoporosis, which resulted in the fall causing her hip to fracture. When she returned home, her fear of falling reduced her ability to regain muscle strength and mobility, which in turn made her more vulnerable to further falls.

Question 4.7

Both women describe falling when alone and hitting their head, causing major bruising and bleeding which was frightening as well as painful. They were both examined by ambulance staff before being taken to hospital. They also mention having difficulties being able to get up again after falling, and they have both had subsequent falls in the home. Both speak fondly of Patrick and how much they enjoyed attending the exercise classes. They both found that the classes lifted their spirits in addition to any improvements the exercises made to their physical coordination at the time; being able to talk to others in similar circumstances was supportive. The first woman looks sad when she says she misses the classes because she could talk to Patrick about anything she had on her mind; the second woman is still going because the classes help her to cope with her situation, even though they aren't really helping her physical mobility any more (in fact this is deteriorating and she needs all the mobility aids that she didn't think she needed at the outset). Both women refer to their anxiety about falling again and their frustration at not being able to go out with confidence, or even get about their homes easily.

Question 5.1

The extracellular matrix in undamaged tissue is made from proteins such as collagen (Chapter 3) which provides much of the structure and function for the tissue and supports the cells within it. Fibrin is sometimes referred to as being a temporary extracellular matrix since it functions to support the cells that migrate into a damaged area (just like the cell support function of normal extracellular matrix), but it is then replaced with more appropriate 'permanent' extracellular matrix proteins. Fibrin is therefore like the scaffolding on a building site – it provides a temporary support while the final building blocks are being arranged.

Question 5.2

Bones generally heal more effectively than tendons because repair in these tissues depends on the presence of cells and an adequate blood supply. Bones have a good blood supply and are populated with cells that make new bone. Tendons, on the other hand, have a poor blood supply and fewer cells, so repair is less effective. In terms of functionality, if bones are realigned and immobilised adequately for repair to occur, then full function can be restored (repaired bone tissue remodels in response to mechanical forces). Tendon repair is less effective (e.g. repaired tendons are usually less elastic and so susceptible to further damage). In addition, fibrosis may cause adhesions between tendons and surrounding tissues, which can damage function.

Question 5.3

Stem cells can divide to produce daughter cells that can become a wide range of specialist cell types. During repair, stem cells resident in the body produce new cells to repopulate areas of damage (e.g. stem cells in damaged bones produce new osteoblasts, which make new bone tissue). Whilst stem cell therapy technology is relatively new, the potential advantages include the ability of stem cells to replenish themselves. This would overcome limitations in the amount of donor tissue available for grafting and if a person's own stem cells were used they would not trigger an immune response. It may also be possible for *regeneration* rather than *repair* to be achieved.

Question 6.1

Poorer people can be disproportionately affected by trauma because often the person who is injured or killed contributed a large percentage of the family's income. The loss of this income, and the cost of medical care for someone who is injured are rarely covered by insurance, so poorer families can be rendered destitute.

Question 6.2

In an office or library a filing system is a method of making it easy to retrieve information when it is wanted. It might be stored alphabetically, by subject, or author, etc. In the human brain the hippocampus is the region that usually manages the storage and retrieval process, somewhat like a very complex filing system. During times of intense fear the amygdala performs a similar role, although its storage system seems to be less 'well behaved' than the system associated with the hippocampus. With the amygdala it is as if books keep falling off shelves, even when you don't want to read them!

Question 6.3

(a) Symptoms that would have led to Jackie being diagnosed as having PTSD include the following: flashbacks that were triggered by events that reminded her of the scene (fireworks); severe symptoms that lasted for longer than a month; her ordinary memory had become very confused.

(b) Jackie had a terrifying experience with an explosion, darkness, smoke and screams; she thought she herself might die; she became aware that others had died; she witnessed horrific injuries in other people.

(c) Jackie relived the events as calmly as possible, so that she could think about them without becoming distressed.

Comments on the Activities

Activity 1.1

Ways of preventing traffic accidents include: better design of roads and traffic control systems, enforcement of traffic laws, public education about road safety, proper safety inspection of cars and stopping cars that fail their safety inspections in developed countries being exported for sale in developing countries.

Ways of reducing the extent of deaths and injuries when accidents occur include enforcing the wearing of seat belts, and the provision of ambulance services with well-trained staff.

REFERENCES

Barraclough, N. (2006) *First Aid Made Easy*, Bradford, First on Scene Training Services.

Bryant, R. A., Guthrie, R. M. and Moulds, M. L. (2003) 'Hypnotizability and posttraumatic stress disorder: a prospective study', *International Journal of Clinical and Experimental Hypnosis*, vol. 51, pp. 382–389.

Carter, C. (2005) 'The use of hypnosis in the treatment of PTSD', *Australian Journal of Clinical and Experimental Hypnosis*, vol. 33, pp. 82–92.

Concha-Barrientos, M., Nelson, D. I., Fingerhut, M., Driscoll, T. and Leigh, J. (2005) 'The global burden due to occupational injury', *American Journal of Industrial Medicine*, vol. 48, pp. 470–481.

Conway, M. A. and Pleydell-Pearce, C. W. (2000) 'The construction of autobiographical memories in the self memory system', *Psychological Review*, vol. 107, pp. 261–288.

Department of Health (2006) *A New Ambition for Old Age: Next Steps in Implementing the National Service Framework for Older People.*

Diagnostic and Statistical Manual of Mental Disorders (4th edn) (1994), Washington DC, American Psychiatric Association.

Ehlers, A. and Clark, D. M. (2000) 'A cognitive model of posttraumatic stress disorder', *Behaviour Research and Therapy*, vol. 38, pp. 319–345.

Felmingham, K., Kemp, A., Williams, L., Das, P., Hughes, G., Peduto, A. and Bryant, R. (2007) 'Changes in anterior cingulate and amygdala after cognitive behaviour therapy of posttraumatic stress disorder', *Psychological Science*, vol. 18, pp. 127–129.

Flynn, J. M. (1998) 'Current treatment options for pediatric femur fractures', *The University of Pennsylvania Orthopaedic Journal*, vol. 11, pp. 27–35.

Ghaffar, A., Hyder, A. A. and Masud, T. I. (2004) 'The burden of road traffic injuries in developing countries: the 1st national injury survey of Pakistan', *Public Health*, vol. 118, no. 3, pp. 211–217.

Global Burden of Disease Project (2002) Statistical Annex. Available from http://www.who.int/healthinfo/statistics/gbdwhoregionmortality2002.xls (Accessed 30 October 2007)

Global Road Safety Partnership (2004) *Impact of Road Crashes on the Poor: Research note,* GRSP, Geneva. Available from http://www.grsproadsafety.org/themes/default/pdfs/The%20Poor_final%20final%20report.pdf (Accessed 30 October 2007)

Halliday, T. and Davey, B. (eds) (2007) *Water and Health in an Overcrowded World*, Oxford, Oxford University Press.

Hauer, K., Becker, C., Lindemann, U. and Beyer, N. (2006) 'Effectiveness of physical training on motor performance and fall prevention in cognitively impaired older persons: a systematic review', *American Journal of Physical Medicine and Rehabilitation*, vol. 85, pp. 847–857.

Heise, L., Ellsberg, M. and Gottemoeller, M. (1999) *Ending Violence Against Women*, population reports vol. 27, no. 4, Baltimore, Johns Hopkins University, School of Public Health.

Kerr, J. B. (1999) *Atlas of Functional Histology*, Mosby.

La Grow, S. J., Robertson, M. C., Campbell, A. J., Glarke, G. A. and Kerse, N. M. (2006) Reducing hazard related falls in people 75 years and older with significant visual impairment: how did a successful program work', *Injury Prevention*, vol. 12, pp. 296–301.

Lowe, J. S. et al. (2006) *Wheater's Functional Histology* (5th edn), Churchill Livingstone

Magariños, A. M., García Verdugo, J. M. and McEwen, B. S. (1997) 'Chronic stress alters synaptic terminal structure in hippocampus', *Proceedings of the National Academy of Sciences*, vol. 94, pp. 14002–14008.

Maguire, E. A., Gadian, D. G., Johnsrude, I. S., Good, C. D., Ashburner, J., Frackowiak, R. S. J. and Frith, C. D. (2000) 'Navigation-related structural change in the hippocampi of taxi drivers', *Proceedings of the National Academy of Sciences*, vol. 97, pp. 4398–4403.

Midgley, C. (ed.) (2008) *Chronic Obstructive Pulmonary Disease: A Forgotten Killer*, Oxford, Oxford University Press.

Mock, C., Joshipura, M. and Goosen, J. (2004) 'Global strengthening of care for the injured', *Bulletin of the World Health Organization*, vol. 82, no. 4, p. 241.

Nantulya, V. M. and Reich, M. R. (2002) 'The neglected epidemic: road traffic injuries in developing countries', *British Medical Journal*, vol. 24, pp. 1139–1141.

NICE (2004) [online] Clinical guideline for the assessment and prevention of falls in older people. Available from: www.nice.org.uk/CG021 (Accessed 5 September 2007)

Organisation of Economic Cooperation and Development (2005) *Health at a Glance: OECD Indicators 2005,* Organisation for Economic Cooperation and Development.

Pathy, M. S. J., Sinclair, A. J. and Morley, J. E. (eds) (2006) *Principles and Practice of Geriatric Medicine* (4th edn), Wiley.

Peden, M., Scurfield, R., Sleet, D., Mohan, D., Hyder, A. A., Jarawan, E. and Mathers, C. (eds) (2004) *World Report on Road Traffic Injury Prevention*, Geneva, WHO.

Rahman, A. K. M. F. (2004) 'The burden of road traffic injuries in South Asia: a commentary', *Journal of the College of Physicians and Surgeons of Pakistan*, vol. 14, no. 12, pp. 707–708.

Rauch, S. L., Whalen, P. J., Shin, L. M., McInerney, S. C., Macklin, M. L., Lasko, N. B., Orr, S. P. and Pitman, R. K (2000) 'Exaggerated amygdala response to masked facial stimuli in posttraumatic stress disorder: a functional MRI study', *Biological Psychiatry*, vol. 47, pp. 769–776.

Rubenstein, L. Z. (2006) 'Falls in older people: epidemiology, risk factors and strategies for prevention', *Age and Ageing*, vol. 35, supp. 2, pp.ii37–ii41.

Seventh report of the Joint National Committee on Prevention, Detection, Evaluation, and Treatment of High Blood Pressure (JNC 7), NIH Publication No. 03-5233, May 2003.

Smart, L. E. (ed.) (2007) *Alcohol and Human Health*, Oxford, Oxford University Press.

Stone, K. L., Ewing, S. K., Lui, L., Ensrud, K. E., Ancoli-Israel, S., Bauer, D. C., Cauley, J. A., Hillier, T. A. and Cummings, S. R. (2006) 'Self-reported sleep and nap habits and risk of falls and fractures in older women: the study of osteoporotic fractures', *Journal of the American Geriatrics Society*, vol. 54, pp. 1177–1183.

Strickland, J. W. (2000) 'Development of flexor tendon surgery: twenty-five years of progress', *Journal of Hand Surgery*, vol. 25A, pp. 214–235.

Toates, F. (ed.) (2007) *Pain*, Oxford, Oxford University Press.

UNIFEM (2002) *Violence Against Women Around the World: Everyday Acts, Innovative Solutions*, New York, United Nations Development Fund for Women.

van Wynsberghe, D., Noback, C. R and Carola, R. (1995) *Human Anatomy and Physiology* (3rd edn), McGraw-Hill Inc.

Watts, C. and Zimmerman, C. (2002) 'Violence against women: global scope and magnitude', *The Lancet*, vol. 359, pp. 1232–1237.

Whooley, M. A., Kip, K. E., Cauler, J. A., Ensrud, K. E., Nevitt, M. C. and Browner, W. S. (1999) 'Depression, falls, and risk of fracture in older women', *Archives of Internal Medicine*, vol. 159, pp. 484–490.

World Health Organization (2002) *The Injury Chart Book*, Geneva, WHO.

Yardley, L., Bishop, P. L., Beyer, N. et al. (2006) 'Older people's views of falls – prevention interventions in six European countries. *The Gerontologist*, vol. 46, pp. 650–660.

Zafar, H., Rehmani, R., Raja, A. J., Ali, A. and Ahmed, M. (2002) 'Registry based trauma outcome: perspective of a developing country', *Emergency Medicine Journal*, vol. 19, pp. 391–394.

Further reading

Driscoll, P., Skinner, D. and Earlam, R. (eds) (1999) *ABC of Major Trauma*, London, BMJ Books.

Primal Pictures, 3D Model of Human Anatomy. Available from: http://www.primalpictures.co.uk [An interactive human anatomy resource.]

Sambrook, P., Schrieber, L., Taylor, T. and Ellis, A. (eds) (2001) *The Musculoskeletal System*, London, Churchill Livingstone.

Standring, S. (ed.) (2004) *Gray's Anatomy* (39th edn), London, Churchill Livingstone.

Young, B. and Heath, J. W. (eds) (2006) *Wheater's Functional Histology* (5th edn), London, Churchill Livingstone.

Useful websites, maintained by the OU Library through the ROUTES system (see 'About this book')

http://www.who.int/violence_injury_prevention/en/ [WHO website on violence and injury prevention.]

http://www.sja.org.uk/sja/first-aid-advice.aspx [St John Ambulance website.]

http://www.nice.org.uk/guidance/index.jsp?action=byID&r=true&o=10956 [NICE clinical guidelines on the assessment and prevention of falls in older people.]

http://www.bmj.com/cgi/content/full/333/7558/53 [*British Medical Journal* Editorial on 'Death and injury on roads'.]

ACKNOWLEDGEMENTS

Grateful acknowledgement is made to the following sources for permission to reproduce material in this book.

Figures

Figures 1.1, 1.3 and 1.12: Peden, M. et al. (2004) *World Report on Road Traffic Injury Prevention*, World Health Organization and The World Bank; Figure 1.2: World Health Organization; Figures 1.4 and 1.8: World Health Organization (2002) *The Injury Chart Book*, World Health Organization; Figure 1.5: © Ralph Henning/Alamy; Figure 1.6: Mark Henley/Panos Pictures; Figure 1.7: *Health at a Glance: OECD Indicators 2005*, OECD Publishing; Figure 1.9: Aeron-Thomas, A. et al. (2004) *Impact of Road Crashes on the Poor*, Global Road Safety Partnership; Figure 1.10: Adnan Ali/AP/PA Photos; Figure 1.11: Dr A. rehman Alvi/Flickr Photo Sharing;

Figure 2.2: Leonid Smirnov/iStockphoto; Figure 2.6: van Wynsberghe, D., Noback, C. R. and Carola, R. (1995) *Human Anatomy and Physiology*, 3rd edn, McGraw-Hill Inc.; Figure 2.7: Barraclough N. (2006) 'Effects of blood loss', *First Aid Made Easy*, 4th edn, First on Scene Training Limited;

Figure 3.3a: Vicky Taylor with thanks to the Mulberry Day Nursery at the Open University; Figure 3.5: Kerr, J. B. (1999) *Atlas of Functional Histology*, Elsevier Science; Figure 3.8: Copyright 2004 Symmation LLC; Figure 3.9: United States Air Force; Figure 3.10: © Copyright 1999–2007 International Osteoporosis Foundation; Figure 3.15: Strickland J. W. (2000) 'The function of the finger flexor tendon puller system', *25th Anniversary Presentation: Development of Flexor Tendon Surgery: Twenty Five Years of Progress*, American Society for Surgery of the Hand; Figure 3.18: Lowe, J. S. et al. (2006) *Wheater's Functional Histology*, 5th edn, Churchill Livingstone; Figure 3.23: TRL Ltd/Science Photo Library; Figure 3.25: James Phillips;

Figure 4.1a: Bates, Custom Medical Stock Photo/Science Photo Library; Figure 4.1b: Du Cane Medical Imaging Ltd/Science Photo Library; Figures 4.1c and 4.12c: © Medical-on-Line/Alamy; Figure 4.1d: Princess Margaret Rose Orthopaedic Hospital/Science Photo Library; Figure 4.1e: James Stevenson/ Science Photo Library; Figure 4.2a: American Academy of Orthopaedic Surgeons; Figure 4.2b: Flynn, J. M. (1998) 'Current treatment options for pediatric femur fractures', *University of Pennsylvania Orthopaedic Journal*, vol. 11, Spring, University of Pennsylvania; Figure 4.3: Phillip Parkinson, Leeds Teaching Hospital NHS Trust; Figure 4.4: Radiological Society of North America; Figure 4.5: Phototake Inc./Photolibrary; Figure 4.6: Johanna Pichowski; Figures 4.10 and 4.12a: © Robert Destefano/Alamy; Figure 4.12b: LearningRadiology.com; Figure 4.12d: © Phototake Inc./Alamy;

Figures 5.1, 5.4 and 5.7: Erik Walbeehm; Figure 5.3: Mercy Ships UK;

Figure 6.1: Martin Roemers/Panos Pictures.

We acknowledge the assistance of Jon Golding in the development of Figure 5.6.

Tables

Table 2.2: Barraclough N. (2006) 'Effects of blood loss', *First Aid Made Easy*, 4th edn, First on Scene Training Limited;

Table 6.1: Aeron-Thomas, A. et al. (2004) *Impact of Road Crashes on the Poor*, Global Road Safety Partnership.

Every effort has been made to contact copyright holders. If any have been inadvertently overlooked the publishers will be pleased to make the necessary arrangements at the first opportunity.

INDEX

Entries and page numbers in **bold type** refer to key words which are printed in **bold** in the text. Indexed information on pages indicated by *italics* is carried mainly or wholly in a figure or a table.

Introducing Health Sciences: A Case Study Approach

Series editor: Basiro Davey

Seven case studies on major topics in global public health are the subject of this multidisciplinary series of books, each with its own animations, videos and learning activities on DVD. They focus on: access to clean water in an overcrowded and polluted world; the integration of psychological and biological approaches to pain; alcohol consumption and its effects on the body; the science, risks and benefits of mammography screening for early breast cancer; chronic lung disease due to smoke pollution – a forgotten cause of millions of deaths worldwide; traffic-related injuries, tissue repair and recovery; and the causes and consequences of visual impairment in developed and developing countries. Each topic integrates biology, chemistry, physics and psychology with health statistics and social studies to illuminate the causes of disease and disability, their impacts on individuals and societies and the science underlying common treatments. These case studies will be of value to anyone who is, or wants to be, working in a health-related occupation where scientific knowledge could enhance your prospects. If you have a wide-ranging interest in human sciences and want to learn more about global health issues and statistics, how the body works and the scientific rationale for screening procedures and treatments, this series is for you.

Titles in this series

Water and Health in an Overcrowded World, edited by Tim Halliday and Basiro Davey

Pain, edited by Frederick Toates

Alcohol and Human Health, edited by Lesley Smart

Screening for Breast Cancer, edited by Elizabeth Parvin

Chronic Obstructive Pulmonary Disease: A Forgotten Killer, edited by Carol Midgley

Trauma, Repair and Recovery, edited by James Phillips

Visual Impairment: A Global View, edited by Heather McLannahan

Trauma, Repair and
Recovery

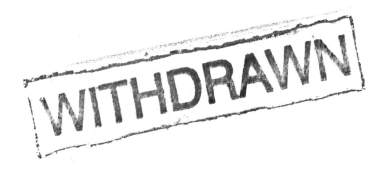